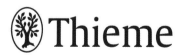

Dr. Vodder's Manual Lymph Drainage

A Practical Guide

Second Edition

Professor Hildegard Wittlinger
Founder, Lymphedema Clinic Wittlinger
Director, Dr. Vodder Academy
Walchsee, Austria

Dieter Wittlinger, PT
CEO, Wittlinger Therapy Center
Lymphedema Clinic Wittlinger
Dr. Vodder Academy
Walchsee, Austria

Andreas Wittlinger, PT
Director of Therapy Department
Lymphedema Clinic Wittlinger
Director, Dr. Vodder Academy
CEO, Dr. Vodder Academy International
Walchsee, Austria

Maria Wittlinger, MT
Director, Lymphedema Clinic Wittlinger
Director, Dr. Vodder Academy
Walchsee, Austria

204 illustrations

Thieme
Stuttgart • New York • Delhi • Rio de Janeiro

Library of Congress Cataloging-in-Publication Data

Names: Wittlinger, Hildegard, author. | Wittlinger, Dieter, author. | Wittlinger, Andreas, author. | Wittlinger, Maria, author.

Title: Dr. Vodder's manual lymph drainage: a practical guide / Hildegard Wittlinger, Dieter Wittlinger, Andreas Wittlinger, Maria Wittlinger.

Other titles: Manuelle Lymphdrainage nach Dr. Vodder. English. | Manual lymph drainage

Description: Second edition. | Stuttgart; New York : Thieme, [2019] | Preceded by Dr. Vodder's manual lymph drainage/Hildegard Wittlinger... [et al. ; translator, Ruth Gutberlet; illustrator, Emil Wolfgang Hanns]. 2011. | Translation of: Manuelle Lymphdrainage nach Dr. Vodder. 2. Aufl. 2016. | Includes bibliographical references and index. |

Identifiers: LCCN 2018038902 (print) | LCCN 2018041066 (ebook) | ISBN 9783132411470 () | ISBN 9783132411449 (softcover) | ISBN 9783132411470 (e-book)

Subjects: | MESH: Lymphedema--therapy | Manual Lymphatic Drainage--methods | Lymphatic System-physiology | Atlases

Classification: LCC RM723.L96 (ebook) | LCC RM723.L96 (print) | NLM WH 17 | DDC 616.4/20622--dc23

LC record available at https://lccn.loc.gov/2018038902

This book is an authorized translation of the 2nd German edition published and copyrighted 2016 by Georg Thieme Verlag, Stuttgart.
Title of the German edition: Manuelle Lymphdrainage nach Dr. Vodder

Translator: Ruth Gutberlet

Illustrators: Emil Wolfgang Hanns, Schriesheim, Germany; Karin Baum, Paphos, Cyprus; Helmut Holtermann, Dannenberg, Germany

1st Czech 2013

1st Japanese 2012

1st Portuguese (Brazil) 2013

1st Spanish 2012

© 2019 Georg Thieme Verlag KG
Thieme Publishers Stuttgart
Rüdigerstrasse 14, 70469 Stuttgart, Germany
+49 [0]711 8931 421, customerservice@thieme.de

Thieme Publishers New York
333 Seventh Avenue, New York, NY 10001, USA
+1-800-782-3488, customerservice@thieme.com

Thieme Publishers Delhi
A-12, Second Floor, Sector-2, Noida-201301
Uttar Pradesh, India
+91 120 45 566 00, customerservice@thieme.in

Thieme Publishers Rio, Thieme Publicações Ltda.
Edifício Rodolpho de Paoli, 25º andar
Av. Nilo Peçanha, 50 – Sala 2508
Rio de Janeiro 20020-906 Brasil
+55 21 3172 2297 / +55 21 3172 1896

Cover design: Thieme Publishing Group
Typesetting by DiTech Process Solutions, India

Printed in Germany by Aprinta Druck GmbH 5 4 3

ISBN 978-3-13-241144-9

Also available as an e-book:
eISBN 978-3-13-241147-0

Important note: Medicine is an ever-changing science undergoing continual development. Research and clinical experience are continually expanding our knowledge, in particular our knowledge of proper treatment and drug therapy. Insofar as this book mentions any dosage or application, readers may rest assured that the authors, editors, and publishers have made every effort to ensure that such references are in accordance with **the state of knowledge at the time of production of the book**.

Nevertheless, this does not involve, imply, or express any guarantee or responsibility on the part of the publishers in respect to any dosage instructions and forms of applications stated in the book. **Every user is requested to examine carefully** the manufacturers' leaflets accompanying each drug and to check, if necessary in consultation with a physician or specialist, whether the dosage schedules mentioned therein or the contraindications stated by the manufacturers differ from the statements made in the present book. Such examination is particularly important with drugs that are either rarely used or have been newly released on the market. Every dosage schedule or every form of application used is entirely at the user's own risk and responsibility. The authors and publishers request every user to report to the publishers any discrepancies or inaccuracies noticed. If errors in this work are found after publication, errata will be posted at www.thieme.com on the product description page.

Some of the product names, patents, and registered designs referred to in this book are in fact registered trademarks or proprietary names even though specific reference to this fact is not always made in the text. Therefore, the appearance of a name without designation as proprietary is not to be construed as a representation by the publisher that it is in the public domain.

Contents

Preface

The content of this second edition was revised. The latest scientific findings of fundamental research in lymphology were implemented, for example, the evidence of lymph vessels in the meninges of mice.

As practitioners of this method, we must ask ourselves what clinical relevance these little steps that are made in fundamental research provide.

As a matter of fact—at least in Austria—the governing body of social security compiles metastudies, which keep questioning the clinical efficiency of manual lymph drainage and combined decongestive therapy. These metastudies keep talking about the small amount of evidence of the efficiency of manual lymph drainage. Further studies need to focus on proving and substantiating that manual lymph drainage therapy is an effective therapy. Only then medicine would be open to recognizing the importance of the method and accepting its effectiveness. Therapists could then count on continuous prescriptions for manual lymph drainage and would be able to provide proof of its effectiveness. The therapists' problem is that MDs know little about the lymph pathways of the skin vessel system and how Vodder's manual lymph drainage achieves its results by influencing the lymph vessel system of the skin.

Nothing has changed in regard to the practical aspects and execution of Dr. Vodder's manual lymph drainage as a whole-body treatment or in combination with physical decongestion therapy. Vodder's techniques are explained to perfection and must be executed precisely in order to achieve the established and desired results.

For the past 50 years, it has been a well-known fact (based on scientific research and proof) that a hastened execution of the techniques or an increased pressure will cause spasms in the lymph vessels. Vodder too emphasized this in his teachings and I vividly remember his lectures. I hope the therapists, who will use this book complementary to their studies, will truly enjoy this technique and recognize manual lymph drainage as a valuable addition to their therapeutic options.

I dedicate this book to my sons Dieter and Andreas as well as to Dieter's wife Maria. They truthfully carry on Vodder's life's work and the enthusiasm that their father had for this method.

Hildegard Wittlinger
Walchsee, Austria

Spring 2019

Part I

Theoretical Basics of Manual Lymph Drainage

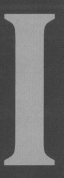

1 Anatomy and Physiology of the Circulation of Blood

1.1 Blood

Blood can be regarded as a liquid tissue. It circulates in the body, driven by a pump, the heart. Our blood accounts for 7 to 8% of our body weight, which in a person of 70 kg (154 lb) body weight amounts to about 4.5 to 6 L of blood. Blood is made up of **blood plasma** and **blood** **cells** (erythrocytes, leukocytes, and thrombocytes; ►**Fig. 1.1**).

Red blood cells (erythrocytes) develop like all other blood cells from pluripotent stem cells in the bone marrow (►**Fig. 1.2**). Erythrocytes contain hemoglobin, which transports oxygen. They are not motile (i.e., they cannot move on their own), but are carried along in the bloodstream.

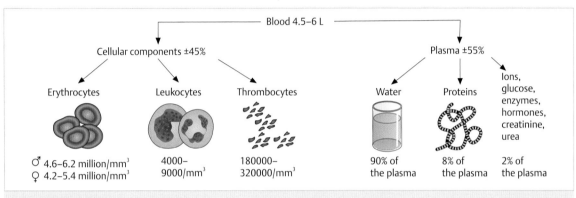

Fig. 1.1 Solid and liquid blood components.

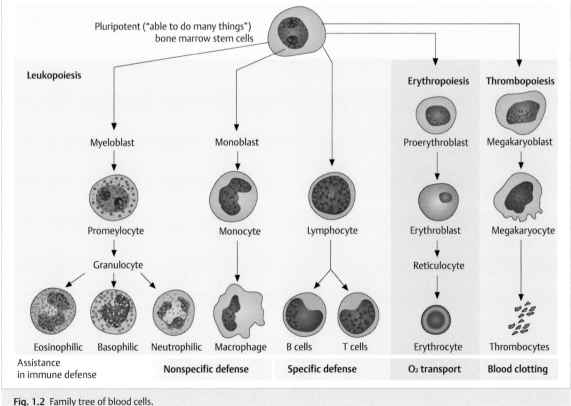

Fig. 1.2 Family tree of blood cells.

White blood cells (leukocytes) include granulocytes (neutrophilic, basophilic, and eosinophilic), lymphocytes, plasma cells, and monocytes.

Thrombocytes are blood platelets, which play an important part in blood coagulation.

Blood plasma contains dissolved organic and inorganic molecules. Albumins make up the majority of **plasma proteins**. They are metabolized in the liver and have a role as transporters, for example, of hormones. Like all plasma proteins, albumins are water soluble and are thus responsible for the colloid osmotic pressure. The immunoglobulins (also called antibodies) are the molecular front of the body's defense system. They are released into the blood by certain lymphocytes, called plasma cells.

Both blood and lymph contain **fibrinogen**, which has a role in coagulation. Examples of organic substances found in blood are lipids, lipid–protein compounds (lipoproteins), hormones, vitamins, amino acids, and bile pigments. "Organic substances" is the name given collectively to all molecules containing the carbon atom C, except for CO (carbon monoxide) and CO_2 (carbon dioxide).

Examples of inorganic substances are phosphate, iodine (I), iron (Fe), potassium (K), and sodium (Na).

The main task of blood is as a transporter. Oxygen is carried from the lungs directly to all tissues via the red blood corpuscles (erythrocytes), and carbon dioxide is carried back from the tissues to the lungs. The only structures excluded from this direct exchange are joint cartilage, a small section of the bone–tendon connection, and parts of the intervertebral disk. In addition, as a liquid medium, the bloodstream transports nutrients from the intestines to the tissues and metabolic waste to the organs of excretion.

1.1.1 Red Blood Cells (Erythrocytes)

Erythrocytes, which are non-nucleated, make up 99% of the corpuscular components of the blood. Their function is to transport oxygen, which bonds in the cell, to hemoglobin, the ferrous blood pigment.

Erythrocytes are formed in the bone marrow and have a life cycle of 120 days. They are broken down in the spleen. At maturity, they are 6 to 7 μm in size, which means they are larger than the diameter of the capillaries. Because they cannot move on their own, they have to be very pliable so that they can be pushed through the capillaries (▶**Fig. 1.3**).

1.1.2 White Blood Cells (Leukocytes)

Leukocytes are not a uniform group of cells. Their three main groups comprise such differing cells as lymphocytes, granulocytes, and monocytes. **Q 50**

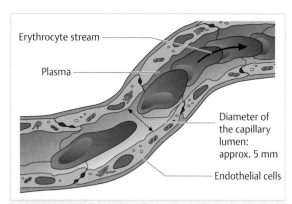

Fig. 1.3 Deformation of red blood cells as they pass through capillaries.

Labels: Erythrocyte stream; Plasma; Diameter of the capillary lumen: approx. 5 mm; Endothelial cells

Granulocytes, which are nonspecific defense cells, make up 60% of leukocytes. They are divided into three groups (▶**Fig. 1.4a–c**):
- Neutrophilic granulocytes (95%).
- Eosinophilic granulocytes (3%).
- Basophilic granulocytes (2%).

With a diameter of 10 to 17 μm, they are considerably larger than the erythrocytes. Granulocytes remain in the blood only for a short period of time, moving on from there to the tissues, especially the mucous membranes, where they fulfill their defense function by destroying bacteria through phagocytosis.

Approximately 30% of white blood cells are lymphocytes. They are 7 to 12 μm in diameter, between erythrocytes and granulocytes in size. Only 4% of lymphocytes circulate in the blood. Most of them are to be found in the lymphatic organs: spleen, thymus, lymphatic intestinal tissue, and lymph nodes.

Lymphocytes are subdivided into two groups: **T lymphocytes**, which are formed in the thymus, and **B lymphocytes**, formed in the bone marrow. These two groups have reciprocal effects. Certain T cells, the T helper cells, can stimulate B lymphocytes after an antigen has sensitized the latter. These B lymphocytes develop into plasma cells, which specialize in producing antibodies. T suppressor cells inhibit the immune response of B lymphocytes and other T cells. Specialized B lymphocytes represent the body's antigen memory. **Q 39**

Lymphocytes come in contact with an antigen in the lymph node. This contact sensitizes them and causes them to reproduce. They leave the lymph node through the efferent lymph vessels, enter the blood, enter the tissues, and then return to the lymph nodes. Lymphocytes spend most of their lifespan in lymph nodes or other lymphatic tissue and only hours (up to 24) in the blood. **Q 11**

Monocytes remain in the blood for a few days and travel from there to the tissues, where they reside as **macrophages** for months or even years. For this reason,

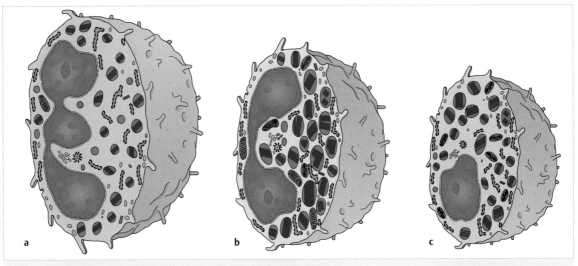

Fig. 1.4 Granulocytes: **(a)** neutrophilic; **(b)** eosinophilic; **(c)** basophilic.

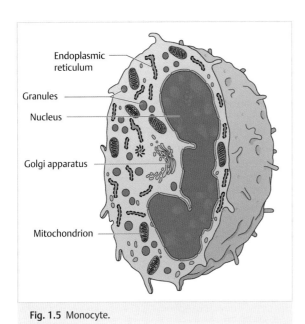

Endoplasmic reticulum

Granules

Nucleus

Golgi apparatus

Mitochondrion

Fig. 1.5 Monocyte.

they are also called histiocytes (from the Greek *histion*, web, tissue). They have a nonspecific part in the defense system: they phagocytose cell debris and antigens. They are quite large (12–20 µm) and possess strong amoeboid motility (▶ **Fig. 1.5**). Q 50

1.1.3 Blood Platelets (Thrombocytes)

Thrombocytes are small, flat, and round non-nucleated cells, 1 to 4 µm in diameter. Their lifespan is 9 to 12 days, during which time they remain in the blood. Their task is controlled coagulation of blood and wound sealing. If the endothelium of the inner vascular wall is damaged, platelets form a thrombus (clump) at the injury site.

Thrombocytes contain serotonin; serotonin causes vasoconstriction, which inhibits blood loss from the damaged vessel and promotes hemostasis.

1.2 Cardiovascular System

The cardiovascular system is made up of the heart and blood vessels. This system supplies oxygen and nutrients to all the cells in the body, and at the same time removes the waste products of metabolism, including carbon dioxide and substances excreted via the urinary system.

In the "greater" **circulatory system**, oxygen-rich blood coming from the lungs is pumped from the left cardiac ventricle, through the aorta, the arteries, the arterioles, and finally the capillaries into the periphery. Passing through the capillary system, the blood moves from the arterial into the venous system. From the venous part of the capillaries, the blood travels to the venules and veins. Propelled by various complementary mechanisms (valves that prevent the venous return), it travels to the right atrium of the heart, into the right ventricle (▶ **Fig. 1.6**). The **muscle pump**, which is activated by any movement of the body, exerts pressure on the veins, particularly in the lower extremities.

The **venous valves** steer the blood in the desired direction. In addition, inspiration creates negative pressure in the thoracic cavity relative to the abdominal cavity, producing a suction that transports the venous blood toward

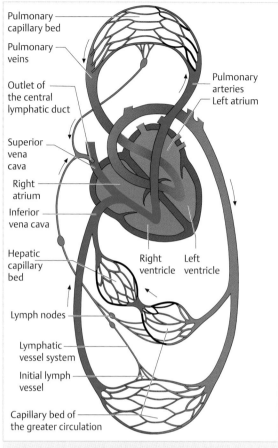

Fig. 1.6 The circulatory system.

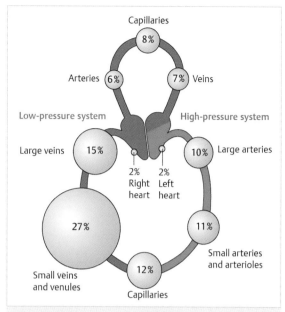

Fig. 1.7 Distribution of the blood volume in the circulatory system.

the heart. The pumping action of the right side of the heart also exerts suction on the vena cava, drawing the blood through this vessel toward the heart. **Q 48**

At this point, the **pulmonary or "lesser" circulation** begins. The right cardiac ventricle pumps the blood into the lungs. Oxygen exchange takes place in the pulmonary alveoli, analogous to the exchange seen in the capillary system. In this case, carbon dioxide (CO_2) is released and oxygen (O_2) is taken up. The oxygen diffuses into the erythrocytes. There it forms a compound with hemoglobin, turning into oxyhemoglobin. The blood travels from the lungs back to the left cardiac ventricle and has come full circle. Thus, the arteries provide the blood flow into the tissues and the veins provide the blood flow out of them (▶ **Fig. 1.7**).

The **blood pressure** is relatively high in the arteries and drops away further down the branches of the system (e.g., the pressure in the brachial artery of the upper arm, where blood pressure is usually taken, is in the range of 120–140/80–90 mm Hg in the healthy adult). Precapillary sphincters lower the pressure in the capillaries to 30 mm Hg. The pressure in the venous system is about

10 to 25 mm Hg; finally, in the veins close to the heart, it drops right down to 2 to 4 mm Hg.

Blood pressure is regulated by complex mechanisms, including the autonomic nervous system, hormones, and even ions. Vasoactive substances include histamine, prostaglandin, serotonin, and epinephrine. The exchange of cell nutrients takes place through the walls of the capillaries, where the flow rate is rather slow. Flow rate, blood pressure, and the diameter (caliber) of the vessels play an important role in metabolic processes. Blood flow is regulated by changes in vascular radius. The flow into the capillary areas is also regulated. At no time are all the capillaries open simultaneously. A large proportion of the blood is stored in the venous system, spleen, and liver. Vascular constriction increases the resistance to blood flow and perfusion decreases.

1.2.1 Arterial System

The arterial wall consists of three layers: the interior vascular endothelium with an elastic membrane (tunica interna or intima); the middle layer with elastic fibers and smooth muscle cells (tunica media); and the outermost connective-tissue layer, which also contains elastic fibers (tunica externa; ▶ **Fig. 1.8**).

This three-layer structure is crucial to maintaining a steady blood flow. The volume of blood expelled with each systole briefly dilates the aorta and the arteries close to the heart. During the diastolic phase, when the heart muscle

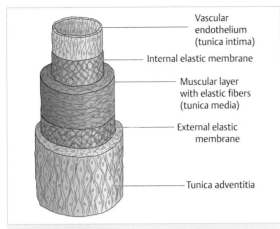

Fig. 1.8 Structure of an arterial wall of the muscular type.

relaxes, these dilated vessels recoil, pushing the blood forward. If the aorta was rigid like a pipe, the blood flow would stop after systole. This mechanism is called the **Windkessel effect**, and it is due to the relatively high percentage of elastic fibers in the vessel wall. Further toward the periphery of the body, the muscular layer is more dominant in the arterial walls. These arteries can actively contract and thus considerably increase the flow resistance of the entire system. For this reason, they are called resistance vessels; they help regulate blood distribution and blood pressure.

The resistance vessels include the arterioles, whose caliber is only 1% that of the arteries. Only about 10% of the blood volume is in the small arteries and arterioles.

The main function of these vessels is to regulate blood flow in the downstream capillary network, which they do by means of their contractility, controlled by the sympathetic nervous system (vasomotion). They therefore have a very strong effect on the function of the body parts that they supply. The precapillary sphincter has two tasks: to regulate (1) capillary blood flow and (2) blood pressure. Increased blood flow will cause active hyperemia. As mentioned earlier, precapillary sphincters can contract if energy needs are low, and send the blood directly into the venous system via an arteriovenous anastomosis. **Q 52**

1.2.2 Capillaries

The capillaries form the transition between the arterial and venous systems. With a diameter of 3 to 8 μm, they are extremely narrow. The walls of the capillaries are made of a single endothelial layer (the endothelial cells are sheathed by the endothelial glycocalyx) and a basement membrane. The wall is semipermeable; that is, depending on its structure (the size of its "windows"), certain substances can selectively pass through. The exchange of substances

is additionally supported by the flow rate in the capillaries, which is very slow. The actual exchange takes place in the capillaries and does so by diffusion, osmosis, and filtration.

1.2.3 Venous System

From the capillaries, the blood travels to the venules, whose walls are only slightly thicker than the capillary walls. They have few muscle fibers and are elastic. From the venules, the venous blood travels to the larger veins, which eventually carry it all the way to the right heart, where it restarts its journey to the lungs for oxygenation. The walls of the **veins** are structured in the same way as the walls of the arteries, but they are considerably thinner; this is adequate because the pressure in the venous system is lower. In the small and middle-sized veins, the inner layers of the walls form small flaps or pouches, called venous valves, which keep the blood from running backward. **Q 48**

The activity of the muscle pump has an important role in maintaining blood flow from the veins back to the heart. When muscles surrounding the veins contract, the blood is pushed toward the heart as long as the venous valves are functioning properly. Thus, the important veins of the legs are located deep in the tissue, where the muscle pump can propel the blood with every movement of the leg. In addition to the deep veins, superficial veins also exist in the legs, forming a close network under the skin. Perforating veins connect the deep veins with the superficial veins. They act as a one-way street and physiologically only allow blood to flow from the surface to the deep layers—not in the other direction.

If the pressure on the venous walls becomes inadequate, the blood can no longer be moved along fast enough and can become stagnant. The veins give way under the internal pressure and dilate, because they have few muscle fibers. As a result, the valves no longer seal the lumen properly, and blood travels backward—increasing the internal pressure even more. This insufficiency of the venous valves leads to **varicose veins** (**varices**).

Approximately 60% of the entire blood volume is located in the venous system; this is why veins are also called **capacitance vessels**. The body can take quite large amounts of blood from this system and send them to any other region if needed, for example, to muscle tissue during physical exercise. **Q 52**

The **lymphatic system** consists of lymph vessels (also called simply "lymphatics"), lymph nodes, and organs, such as tonsils, spleen, thymus, lymphatic mucous membrane tissue, and the tissue of the appendix. Structures lacking lymphatics are epidermis, glandular epithelium, bone marrow, brain, cartilage, nails, lens, and the vitreous body. The last four of these do not contain blood vessels either.

2 Anatomy of Lymph Vessels and Lymph Nodes

The lymphatic system can be divided into a superficial system and a deep system. The superficial (epifascial) system removes the interstitial fluid of the skin. The deep (subfascial) system removes interstitial fluid from muscles, joints, organs, and vessels. The two systems are interconnected via perforating lymph vessels.

The vessels of the deep system empty into the large lymph trunks.

With regard to the lymph system, the skin is divided in sections. Initial lymph vessels (lymph capillaries) drain the lymph-obligatory load of one of the small, overlapping, circular areas of skin (1–3 cm in diameter) into which the entire covering of the body is divided. From the **initial lymph vessel**, the lymph moves to the precollectors. Several adjacent skin areas constitute a skin zone, the **precollectors** of which are interconnected and empty into a common lymph collector. **Collectors** drain lymph from strip like skin zones. Several skin zones together form a **lymph vessel bundle**, also called a **territory**. There are no anastomoses between the bundles, only between collectors within a bundle.

The vessel bundles drain into the lymph node stations (inguinal and axillary), and ultimately into the thoracic duct and the venous angle.

The superficial (epifascial) lymph vessels are spread out like a network and frequently run parallel to the superficial veins. The subfascial lymph vessels of muscles, joints, bones, and organs run with the blood vessels (in the neurovascular sheath) and do not have their own names.

> **Note**
>
> The **lymph-obligatory load** is the name given to all the substances that have to be removed from the interstitium via the lymphatic vascular system. **Q 9**

The lymphatic vascular system is a second drainage system that supports the venous system in removing substances from the interstitium. Because of its particular anatomy, the lymph vessels can absorb and remove all those molecules that are too large or too many to enter the venous system. These substances are called the "lymph-obligatory load" and consist mainly of proteins, long-chain fatty acids, cells and cell debris, and water. Exogenous substances such as viruses, bacteria, coal dust, and glass dust (silica) are also removed in this way. **Q 9**

The lymph from the entire body drains into the subclavian vein at the venous angle (terminus) and travels together with the venous blood into the right heart. Just as in the arterial and venous systems, there is a hierarchy of scale (size) in the channels of the lymphatic system.

> **Note**
>
> *Lymph-obligatory loads:* **Q 10**
> - *Water (also serves transportation).*
> - *Protein.*
> - *Lipids.*
> - *Cells.*
> - *Exogenous substances.*

2.1 Initial Lymph Vessels

Prelymphatics are small channels found in the loose connective tissue. They do not have a vascular structure, but they do carry lymph-obligatory substances.

The initial lymph vessels (also known as lymph sinus, formerly called lymph capillaries) are the smallest vessels and form the beginning of the lymphatic vascular system. The lymph vessels of interest for manual lymph drainage (MLD) are those of the skin. The initial lymph vessels can be found in the entire dermis and drain the lymph-obligatory load from the connective tissue or interstitium.

Initial lymph vessels are reticulated. Some have a blind origin in the tissue. They consist of a single oak-leaf-shaped layer of endothelial cells that connect with adjacent cells. Some overlap at the edges and do not close tightly, so they can open like shutter valves (▶ **Fig. 2.1**). **Q 1, Q 2**

The vessel is surrounded by a basement membrane (fiber network), which is much thinner than the basement membrane of blood capillaries. This reticular fiber network and the anchor filaments, which insert directly at the endothelial cells and the fiber network, are connected to the fibers of the surrounding tissue. When tissue pressure is low, the intercellular openings (open junctions) are closed. When the pressure in the connective tissue changes or more water enters the tissue, tissue pressure rises. The connective tissue swells and the collagen fibers of the connective tissue pull on the fiber network (matrix) and the anchor filaments, creating an opening from the endothelial cells into the initial lymph vessel. Through this opening, water, large molecules, cell debris, and cells can enter the initial lymph vessel. The exact mechanism and process of how the lymph-obligatory load flows into the initial lymph vessel is still not fully understood.

According to Zoeltzer (2003), opening and closing of the open junctions is an active process of the endothelial cell.

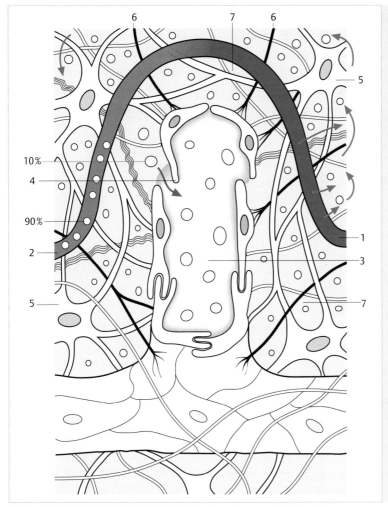

Fig. 2.1 Longitudinal section along a glove-finger-shaped initial lymph vessel with a blind origin in the tissue. 1, arterial limb of capillary; 2, venous limb of capillary; 3, initial lymph vessel; 4, swinging tip of an endothelial cell of the initial lymph vessel allowing influx of interstitial fluid (*arrow* to the left and right of 4); 5, fibrocyte; 6, anchor filaments; 7, intercellular space.

This would indicate a much more complex process than has been assumed so far. Diffusion, osmosis, or suction created through contraction of the deeper lymph vessels are considered to be a part of the mechanism. During influx into the initial lymph vessel, pressure in the vessel increases and pressure in the interstitium correspondingly decreases, while the shutter valves close. The initial lymph vessel is also called a collecting vessel and empties into the precollectors. Precollectors are often closely connected with arteries and their pulsation results in an acceleration of lymph flow. **Q 1, Q 2**

2.2 Precollectors

Initial lymph vessels turn without noticeable transition into precollectors, which pass the collected lymph on to the next vessels (the collectors). In the skin (and also in the mucous membranes), they run vertically into the deep tissues.

The precollectors show similarities to both the smaller and the larger lymph vessels. They have rudimentary valves that determine the direction of flow and also prevent reflux. There are some isolated muscle fibers and openings in the walls that allow them to absorb fluid from the connective tissue.

Precollectors have a transitional character. On the one hand, they are transport vessels and form the link between the initial lymph vessels and the collectors. In addition, though, like the initial lymph vessels they are able to absorb a small amount of lymph-obligatory substances from the interstitium and are therefore also regarded as collecting vessels. The collectors to some extent have a suction effect on the content of the precollectors, which speeds up the transport. As mentioned earlier, this suction can continue to have an effect all the way into the initial lymph vessels. **Q 3, Q 4**

2.3 Lymph Collectors

The lymph collectors are the next size up from the lymph vessels. Along their course from the periphery to the venous angle, lymph nodes are interposed. The wall of the lymph collectors exhibits the classic three-layered structure of the entire vessel system: intima, media, and adventitia.

The **intima** consists of endothelial cells with flaps every 6 to 20 mm. The section between two paired flaps (valves) is called a lymph vessel segment or, to use Mislin's (1984) term, **lymphangion**. The valves control the direction of flow.

The **media** is mainly made up of smooth muscle cells, with a multilayered structure consisting of a medial circular layer and a longitudinal layer. This is a spiral-like plexus that may include several angions. It also contains some thin collagen fibers. The muscles are only found in the middle section between the valves: the valves themselves are without muscles. This gives an impression of constriction at the valves, leading to a "string of pearls" appearance on contrast imaging.

The **adventitia** is the support layer, made of strong collagenous fibers that merge with the extravascular connective tissue. **Q 5**

When the lymph flow increases, the internal pressure rises, the wall of the vessel stretches, and its tension increases. This is the triggering stimulus for the muscle cells of the lymphangion to contract. The contraction drives the lymph proximally, while the distal valves close (▶**Fig. 2.2**).

The lymph flow is also maintained by so-called **auxiliary pumps**. The following factors exert external pressure on the vessels:
- MLD.
- Contraction of skeletal muscles.
- Pulsation of large arteries (subfascially blood vessels always accompany the lymph vessels).

- Increased intestinal peristalsis during MLD.
- Pressure changes in the thorax during respiration that cause intensified contraction of the large lymph trunks and produce a suction effect in the venous angle. **Q 6**

Lymphangions also have their own pulsation, which is independent of internal pressure, with a frequency at rest of four to eight pulsations per minute.

One of the most important auxiliary pumps is **MLD**. The collectors lie in the subcutis, and during Dr. Vodder's MLD they are stretched both lengthways and crossways. Stretching the lymphangions increases the pulsation rate, accelerating the flow of the lymph (Mislin 1984).

Hence, both a large amount of lymph and MLD result in an acceleration of lymph flow. MLD does so through a particular technique. Sympathicolysis is an additional effect of MLD, as described by Hutzschenreuter (1994). It causes dilatation of the lymph collector, which increases the contraction of the lymphangion. **Q 6**

There are also **inhibiting** influences on the lymphangiomotoricity, that is, the lymph flow is slowed down. Those include the following:
- Local anesthesia.
- Excessive external pressure.
- Pain.
- Strong stimulus fluctuations, for example, through temperature or current.
- Sustaining influences: increase of lymph time volume (e.g., via filtration) caused by autonomic regulation. **Q 6**

> ### Note
>
> *When the lymph-obligatory load has been absorbed into the vessels from the connective tissue, and lymphangion motoricity has been increased by MLD, the suction produced by the lymphangions reaches as far as the initial lymph vessels, which then suck in more lymph-obligatory substances. Transport and removal of these are in turn accelerated by the increased lymphangion pulsation rate.*
>
> *The initial lymph vessel is a collecting vessel. It absorbs the lymph-obligatory load into the vessel system.*
>
> *The precollector is both a transport and a collecting vessel. It can both absorb lymph-obligatory load (though only in small amounts) and transport lymph from the initial lymph vessels to the collectors.*
>
> *The collector is called a transport vessel. It maintains the lymph flow and recycles the lymphocytes.* **Q 6**

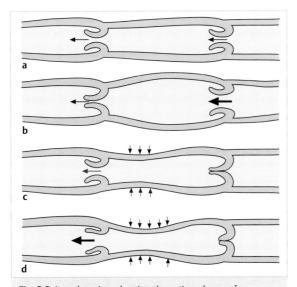

Fig. 2.2 Lymphangion, showing the action phases of lymphatic drainage. **a**, continuous flow in the distal and proximal open flap; **b**, wall distension with more filling from distal; **c**, contraction the angion wall; **d**, subsequent closure of the distal valve and expulsion of the fluid to the proximal direction (according to Pritschow).

2.4 Lymph Nodes

Lymph nodes that are usually found in groups or chains are filtering stations located along the lymph collector paths.

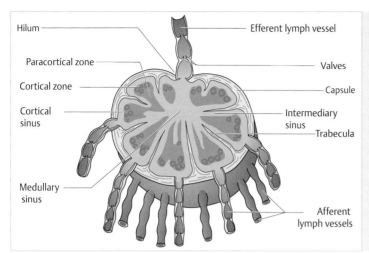

Fig. 2.3 Lymph node.

There are about 600 to 700 lymph nodes in the human body, about 160 of them in the neck region alone. They are mostly bean shaped, with a diameter of 2 to 30 mm, and are surrounded by a connective-tissue capsule that contains some smooth muscle cells (▶ **Fig. 2.3**). However, they can vary considerably in size, shape, and number. Every region of the body has its own group of **regional lymph nodes**. They consist of an internal trabecular framework, which surrounds the lymphatic tissue. Each lymph node has several afferent vessels that enter through the convex side of the capsule and empty into the sinus (marginal, intermediary, and cortical sinus) of the node. One or two lymph vessels exit the capsule at the hilum.

Blood and nerve fiber supply takes place at the hilum. Some lymph vessels may pass the lymph node by. This can be important, in cancer, for example, because it means that metastasis of more centrally located lymph nodes can occur without the regional nodes being involved. **Q 7**

The responsibilities of lymph nodes are manifold. They may be described as biological filters, filtering out everything harmful to the body and rendering it harmless—viruses, bacteria, fungi, and so on. The lymph is cleaned. In the lymph node sinus, antigens (bacteria) are broken down just as they are in the liver.

In addition, lymph is either concentrated upto about 50% or diluted in the lymph nodes, meaning that water is removed, or added, dependent on osmotic pressure differences between lymph and blood.

In the lymph nodes, mature defense cells come into contact with antigens that are being carried in the lymph. Sensitized by contact with an antigen, the lymphocytes in the lymph node are stimulated to divide and a specific defense can get under way. The agglomeration of B lymphocytes in lymph nodes is called **lymph follicle**. At first, they are primary follicles, then after contact with an infectious antigen they become secondary follicles. T lymphocytes (so-called "killer" cells) can also be found in the lymph nodes; they too will become sensitized by contact with an antigen, reproduce, and start to act specifically against that antigen. They are taken up by venules in the lymph nodes, returned to the blood circulation, and then travel back again to the lymph nodes via the lymphatic vessels. **Q 8**

B lymphocytes become plasma cells and form antibodies that are likewise part of the specific defense mechanism against antigens. In addition to initiating antigen defense responses, however, lymph nodes act as a storage place for substances that cannot be excreted by the body, including coal dust, glass dust, and soot. **Q 42**

> **Note**
>
> *Lymph nodes have the following functions:* **Q 8**
> - *Lymph filtration.*
> - *Lymph concentration, if necessary also dilution.*
> - *Activation of the immune system (lymphocyte sensitization).*
> - *Storage place for nondegradable substances.*
> - *Fluid exchange.*

2.5 Lymphatic Trunks

The lymphatic trunks form the final part of the journey for the lymph on its way back into the blood circulation. The thoracic duct, 2 to 4 mm in diameter and 40 cm long in an adult, is the largest lymph vessel, followed by the right lymphatic duct (▶ **Fig. 2.4**). The valves of the thoracic duct are approximately 8 cm apart. They receive the cleansed lymph from the regional lymph nodes. Few lymph nodes are found along the ducts. Their wall structure is typically vascular and pretty much the same as in the lymph collectors, except that the muscular layer is thicker and the valves are further apart.

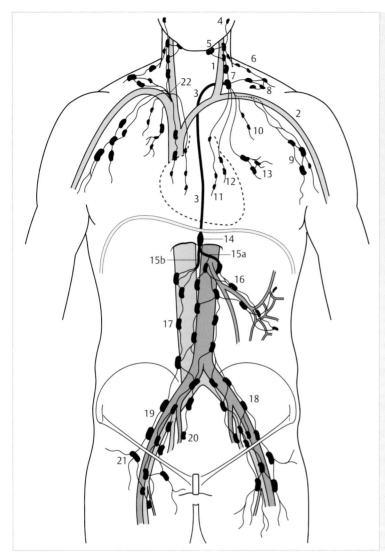

Fig. 2.4 The most important lymphatic trunks and lymph node groups of the body. 1, (left) internal jugular vein; 2, (left) subclavian vein; 3, thoracic duct; 4, parotid nodes; 5, submandibular nodes; 6, concomitant nodes of the accessory nerve; 7, internal jugular nodes with (left) jugular trunk; 8, supraclavicular nodes with (left) supraclavicular trunk; 9, axillary nodes with (left) subclavian trunk; 10, intercostal nodes with (left) intercostal trunk; 11, parasternal nodes with (left) parasternal trunk; 12, anterior mediastinal nodes with (left) anterior mediastinal trunk; 13, tracheobronchial nodes with (left) tracheobronchial trunk; 14, cisterna chyli; 15a, left lumbar trunk; 15b, right lumbar trunk; 16, mesenteric nodes; 17, lumbar nodes; 18, iliac nodes; 19, iliac nodes; 20, iliac nodes; 21, inguinal nodes; 22, right lymphatic duct.

Blood is supplied to the vascular walls through the vasa vasorum, located in the adventitia together with some nerve fibers.

2.5.1 Large Lymphatic Pathways

In the trunk, 11 large lymphatic vessels are found, 5 paired and 1 unpaired:
- Right and left iliac trunks.
- Right and left lumbar trunks.
- Intestinal trunk.
- Right and left jugular trunks.
- Right and left subclavian trunks.
- Right and left bronchomediastinal trunks.

At the level of the navel and the second and third lumbar vertebrae, the right and left lumbar trunks and the intestinal trunk merge and form the cisterna chyli, which turns into the thoracic duct.

The **cisterna chyli** collects lymph from the intestines, abdominal organs, and legs. After a fatty meal, the lymph turns a milklike color due to the fat droplets received from the intestines, hence the name chyle lymph.

The **thoracic duct**, after draining the left side of the body and skin above the diaphragm, left arm, left side of the head, and the entire body below the diaphragm , discharges into the left venous angle, where the subclavian and internal jugular veins join.

The lymph from the right upper body, the right arm, and the right side of the head passes through the right subclavian and jugular trunk (which sometimes join to form the right lymphatic duct) to discharge directly into the right venous angle.

Because the lower body is so far from the venous angles, it needs a large vessel, the thoracic duct, to carry the lymph to the discharging junction. Areas close to the junction can be drained through short single trunks. These trunks discharge into the veins by themselves (primary trunks) or joined in various combinations.

The number of lymph vessels and lymph nodes varies from person to person. What matters is that the lymph-obligatory load can be removed consistently and the lymph nodes are able to perform their function.

Lymph Vessel System of the Skin

Watersheds are notional lines drawn on the basis of the different directions of lymphatic flow. They are located only in the subcutis. In treatment with MLD, the direction of pressure depends on the flow direction of the lymph vessels of the skin, the collector vessels. Watersheds are usually found between two bundles (territories) because very few lymph vessels (cross-connections) exist between the collectors of neighboring bundles (▶ **Fig. 2.5** and ▶ **Fig. 2.6**). In other words, it is an interterritorial area poor in vessels. Under physiological conditions, the direction of drainage for the lymph vessels is divided. Under pathological conditions, reversion of the direction of lymph flow is possible. **Q 16**

The following watersheds are important for MLD:
- Running horizontally across the navel and the second or third lumbar vertebra, dividing the skin into upper and lower body.
- Running vertically along the midline of the body, dividing it into a right and a left half.
- Running along the clavicle and the spine of the scapula, forming a small strip above the shoulders.

Other watersheds exist, but they are not of interest for MLD. **Q 17**

The skin of the body can be divided into four **main quadrants**:
- Right upper quadrant.
- Left upper quadrant.
- Right lower quadrant.
- Left lower quadrant.

The right upper thoracic quadrant drains the lymph of the skin into the lymph nodes of the right axilla. The left upper thoracic quadrant drains into the lymph nodes of the left axilla. **Q 13b**

The lymph of the skin of the lower quadrants is drained into the respective inguinal lymph nodes.

The skin area between the clavicle and scapular spine drains directly into the supraclavicular lymph nodes (in the venous angle).

The **mammary gland** drains to the axilla, to supraclavicular and retrosternal lymph nodes. **Q 15a**

The **skin of the head** is divided into the facial and the posterior skull. The lymph is moved through periauricular, retroauricular, and submandibular lymph nodes, and through occipital lymph nodes along the nuchal line, to the superficial and deep cervical lymph nodes, emptying from there into the venous angle. There are many cross-connections (anastomoses) from one side to the other in the zones of the head. **Q 14e**

Treatment of the neck (in the absence of contraindications, Dr. Vodder's MLD always begins with treatment of the neck) relates to the following sets of lymph nodes:
- Supraclavicular.
- Infraclavicular.
- Along the internal and external jugular vein.
- Along the accessory nerve plexus.

Lymphatic Pathways of the Lower Extremities

The lymphatic vessel system of the lower extremities consists of superficial (epifascial) and deep (subfascial)

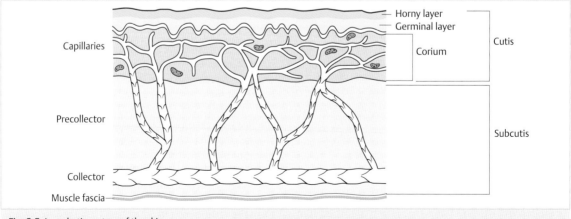

Fig. 2.5 Lymphatic system of the skin.

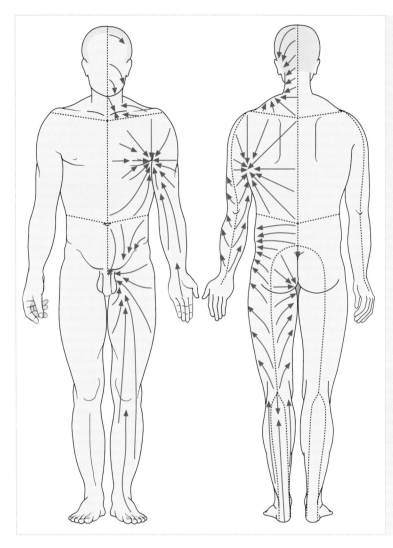

Fig. 2.6 Lymphatic watersheds, lymphatic anastomoses, and lymphatic territories.

lymph vessels (▶**Fig. 2.7**). The superficial vessels absorb approximately 80% of the lymph and the deeper vessels the other 20%. In the lower leg, there are many cross-connections between superficial and deep vessels.

The lymph of the leg drains into the inguinal lymph nodes, both superficial and deep. The superficial inguinal lymph nodes drain to the deeper nodes, which also receive lymph from the deeper lymphatic pathways of the leg.

From there, the lymph travels via the external iliac lymph nodes in the pelvis to the lumbar nodes in the abdomen. Together with the gastrointestinal lymphatic trunk, they join the cisterna chili and actually form it. **Q 15**

The skin of the legs is subdivided as follows:

- *Dorsolateral bundle of the lower leg:* Lymph from the lateral margin of the foot, lateral malleolus, and the medial aspect of the calf is absorbed and drains into the deep lymph nodes in the popliteal space (popliteal nodes) and travels from there along the femur to the deep inguinal lymph nodes.
- *Ventrolateral bundle of the lower leg:* Lymph from the anterior part of the foot and the remaining skin territories of the lower leg is absorbed and drains medially into the long lymph vessels that run ventromedially along the anterior and medial part of the lower leg and the medial part of the knee. They turn into the ventromedial bundle of the upper leg and discharge (epifascially) into the inguinal lymph nodes.

The lymph vessels of the entire back of the leg run ventrally and drain into the ventromedial bundle. The anteromedial bundle contains the longest lymph vessels of the body. Some run without interruption from the foot all the way up to the inguinal lymph nodes and drain into the superficial inguinal lymph nodes. There are "bottlenecks" on the

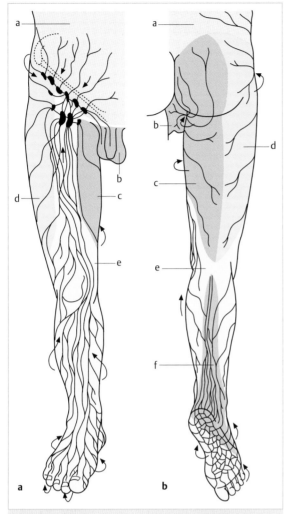

Fig. 2.7 Superficial drainage territories of the lower extremities and the adjacent trunk. The *arrows* indicate the main directions of lymphatic drainage. **(a)** Front (anterior). **(b)** Back (posterior). a, lower trunk territory; b, territory of the outer genitals; c, dorsomedial femoral territory; d, dorsolateral thigh territory; e, territory of the ventromedial bunch; f, territory of dorsolateral bunch.

medial aspect of the knee and at the medial malleolus, that is, the vessels run very close together here.

Cross-connections (anastomoses) exist between the deep and the superficial lymph vessels of the leg. Because of muscular activity, lymph travels from the deep to the superficial vessels. **Q 15c**

In **the lower leg, the deep lymph vessels** run along the anterior and posterior tibial arteries and the fibular arteries. In the upper leg, the deep lymph vessels run along the femoral vessels and empty into the deep inguinal lymph nodes—and sometimes directly into the iliac lymph nodes. **Q 15c**

Some lymph vessels, arising from the popliteal lymph nodes, run along the sciatic nerve. They drain part of the back of the upper leg and empty into the iliac or the lumbar nodes of the abdomen, passing by the inguinal lymph nodes. This is very important in patients with lymph stasis in the inguinal area! **Q 15c**

The lymph of the abdominal wall and the skin of the lumbar region—below the horizontal watershed—drains into the inguinal lymph nodes. **Q 15b**

The **external genitals** also drain their lymph into the inguinal lymph nodes. The lymph from the testicles empties into the lumbar lymph nodes.

> ### Note
>
> *The lymph vessels that run along the sciatic nerve can become very important if the normal drainage pathways of the leg become obstructed, and may function as a circulatory bypass.* **Q 15c**

Lymphatic Pathways of the Upper Extremities

The lymphatics in the arms are both superficial (epifascial) and deep (subfascial; ▶ Fig. 2.8 and ▶ Fig. 2.9). They form a functional unit and are cross-connected. Thus, the lymph runs not just from distal to proximal but also from the superficial to the deep vessels and vice versa.

The lymph of the entire arm is drained to the axillary lymph nodes (lateral and central axillary, subscapular, and pectoral lymph nodes). From there, it is moved through the infraclavicular and supraclavicular lymph nodes into the subclavian trunk and the right and left venous angles. The superficial vessels running along the front of the arm in the subcutaneous connective tissue absorb approximately 80% of the lymph of the entire arm and are hence more important than the deep vessels.

The palmar rete (network) drains the volar part of the hand and fingers. Lymph collectors are located on the lateral aspects of the fingers and the back of the hand. They merge with the ulnar or radial bundle.

The **back of the hand** is almost without subcutaneous fatty tissue, and for this reason, unlike in the palm of the hand with its tight connective tissue, edema can develop easily.

In the **forearm**, a medial bundle and a radial and ulnar bundle are found; they join at the bend of the elbow, where some lymph nodes (superficial cubital lymph nodes) are present, and travel on as the medial bundle of the upper arm to the axillary lymph nodes.

The medial bundle of the **upper arm** runs parallel to the basilic vein and is also called the basilar lymphatic bundle.

The lateral and the posterolateral bundle drain the upper arm and shoulder and discharge the lymph into

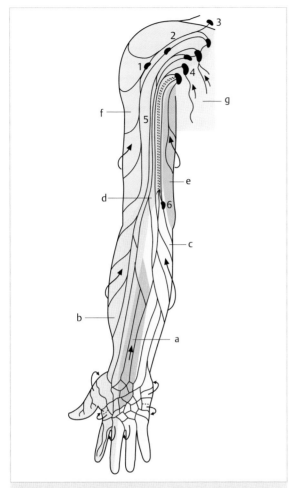

Fig. 2.8 Superficial lymphatic system of the upper extremities, front (palmar). 1, Lnn. deltoideopectoral; 2, lateral upper arm or deltoid bundle; 3, Ln. supraclavicular; 4, Lnn. axillary; 5, median upper arm; 6, Ln. cubital superficial. **a**, middle forearm territory with median forearm bundle; **b**, territory of the radial bundle; **c**, territory of the ulnar bundle; **d**, middle upper arm territory; **e**, dorsomedial upper arm territory; **f**, dorsolateral upper arm shoulder territory; **g**, upper trunk territory.

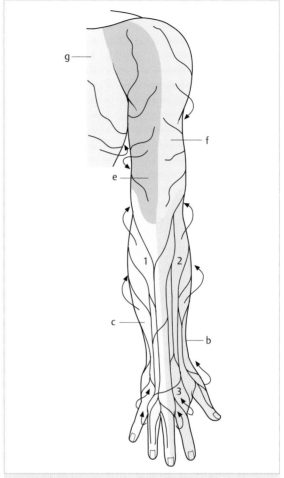

Fig. 2.9 Superficial lymphatic system of the upper extremities, back (posterior). 1, ulnar bundle; 2, radial bundle; 3, transverse collaterals between radial and ulnar hand back collectors; **b**, territory of the radial bundle; **c**, territory ulnar bundle; **e**, dorsomedial upper arm territory; **f**, dorsolateral upper arm and shoulder territory; **g**, upper trunk territory.

the axillary lymph nodes. In some but not all people, a cephalic bundle may emerge from the lateral bundle of the upper arm and travel via the deltoid muscle directly to the supra- or infraclavicular lymph nodes, bypassing the axillary nodes. There is a so-called long type, which has anastomoses to the radial lymphatic bundle of the forearm; the short type does not have these connections.

The cephalic lymph vessel is important when drainage is obstructed in the axilla after lymphadenectomy (surgical removal of lymph nodes) or radiation therapy. **Q 14a**

The anterior and posterior **thoracic walls**—as defined by the aforementioned watersheds—drain the lymph into the right and left axillary lymph nodes. **Q 14b**

The **intercostal lymph vessels** of the back drain into the paravertebral or intercostal lymph nodes, which are located along the spinal column and usually empty into the thoracic duct. **Q 14c**

The **intercostal lymph vessels** of the anterior thorax drain into the parasternal or intercostal lymph nodes and have a runoff to the venous angle and the cisterna chyli. **Q 14c**

2.5.2 Drainage from the Abdomen

From the inguinal lymph nodes, the lymph travels beneath the inguinal ligament into the plexuses and

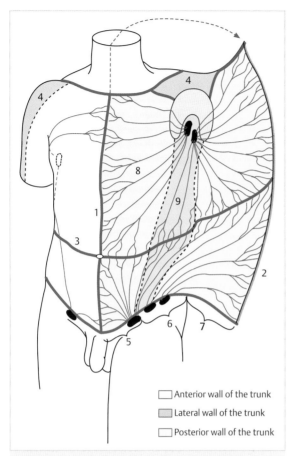

Fig. 2.10 Superficial lymphatic system of the trunk with watersheds and anastomosis. 1, front vertical watershed; 2, rear vertical watershed ("unfolded"); 3, transversal watershed; 4, drainage area of the lateral upper arm bundle; 5, anterior trunk wall; 6, middle hull wall; 7, rear hull wall; 8, interaxillary collaterals; 9, axillo-inguinal collaterals.

Anterior wall of the trunk

Lateral wall of the trunk

Posterior wall of the trunk

nodes of the lesser pelvis—the (paired) iliac lymph nodes, which absorb and remove the lymph from the urogenital organs of the lesser pelvis (urethra, bladder, prostate, pelvic floor, etc.). From the aortic bifurcation, these lymphatic pathways accompany the aorta and the inferior vena cava as the right and left lumbar trunks (again in the form of plexuses) to the cisterna chyli. They drain the lymph of the abdominal organs and, together with the intestinal trunk that joins them coming from the large and small intestines, form the cisterna chyli, from which the thoracic duct originates. After a meal, the lipid content gives the lymph the milklike appearance that gives the cisterna chyli its name. The intestinal lymph is also called chyle lymph. It is removed by various vessels, all of which empty into the cisterna chyli. **Q 15d**

2.5.3 Drainage from the Thorax

The thorax contains four large lymphatic trunks:
- Anterior mediastinal trunk.
- Bronchomediastinal trunk.
- Parasternal trunk.
- Posterior intercostal trunk.

All of these have a right and a left branch. The bronchomediastinal trunks collect the lymph from the lymph nodes located along the aorta, the esophagus, and the lungs. **Q 14c**

> **Note**
>
> *Lymph from the left lower lobe of the lung, the heart, and the right lung is transported to the right venous angle via the right bronchomediastinal trunk and the right lymphatic duct.*

The parasternal trunks receive the lymph from the medial area of the mammary glands and from the intercostal spaces of the anterior thorax, and transport it via the infraclavicular lymph nodes to the venous angle or retrograde to the thoracic duct or the cisterna chyli. The lateral aspect of the mammary glands flows into the axillary. **Q 14c**

The anterior mediastinal trunks receive lymph from organs including the thyroid gland, thymus, and trachea, and empty into the thoracic duct. **Q 14d**

The inflow from the vessels that eventually deliver the lymph to the venous angle varies considerably.

2.5.4 Drainage from the Brain

The brain has no lymph vessels. Neurons are serviced by glial cells, which supply nutrients to the nerve cells and remove metabolic waste. Hence, no lymph-obligatory substances are produced. In the glandular area, where the metabolic exchange rate is high and some of the blood capillaries are fenestrated, lymph-obligatory load is produced; here it is called **prelymph**. With no lymph vessels in either the brain or the spinal cord, there must be other ways for the prelymph to be removed from these regions.

In experiments with injected ink, color particles were found in the cerebrospinal fluid, showing that the lymph-obligatory load can leave the bony skull in this way, from the spinal cord into the venous plexus.

The cranial nerves serve as a "conductor" for the prelymph toward the lamina cribrosa (ethmoid bone).

About 40 to 50% of the prelymph in the brain exits the skull with the olfactory nerve. The nerve fibers run through the sievelike structure of the ethmoid bone. Extracranially, the prelymph is received by the lymph vessels of the nasopharyngeal area, passes the palatal arches, and travels to the deep lymph nodes of the neck. The optic and the vestibulocochlear nerves likewise serve as a "guide track" for the prelymph. Preformed tissue channels of the blood vessels of the brain (the intra-adventitial Virchow–Robin spaces) also exist, which lead the prelymph to the lymphatic pathways of the blood vessel system (carotid artery, vertebral artery, internal jugular artery). **Q 13**

In addition, we would like to quote from Weissleder and Schuchhasrdt (2015): "Experiments provided the following results: it was shown that in mice cerebro-spinal fluid is also drained into the meninges via lymph vessels. Lymph vessel structures were also detected in the human dura. Additional studies in regard to their exact location and further analysis are considered imperative."

2.5.5 Anastomoses

Anastomoses are "inactive" vessels that can be activated when necessary. The activation can be brought about by pressure changes in the lymphatic system caused by stasis (congestion) in the efferent vessels. They can also be opened in the desired direction by MLD. The following anastomoses are important in the treatment of lymphedema:

- Axilloaxillary across the sternum and between the shoulder blades.
- Axilloinguinal, between axillary and inguinal lymph nodes, right and left, or inguinal axillary.
- Suprapubic and across the sacrum.
- Between intercostal vessels and the skin.

Lymph can also be moved across all the watersheds and in all directions in the area of the initial lymph vessels, because of the overlapping skin areas. **Q 43**

> **Note**
>
> *All lymph produced below the navel are ultimately drained by the thoracic duct.*

> **Note**
>
> *When crossing joints, lymph vessels usually run on the medial aspect, rarely along the extensor side. This prevents overextension of the vessels, which could occur if they were on the extensor side.*

All joints are drained through the deep lymphatic system. Drainage begins in the synovial and fibrous membrane of the joint capsule.

3 Physiology of the Lymphatic System, Lymph, and Interstitium

3.1 Loose Connective Tissue

Loose connective tissue plays a huge role in determining the body shape. It does this in conjunction with cartilage and bones, which belong to the more rigid supportive type of connective tissue. The different types of connective tissues are also differentiated through the varying ratio of these components. Connective tissue is divided into three types:

- Mesenchyme, rich in cells (embryonic connective tissue).
- Loose, adipose connective tissue, rich in fibers and cells.
- Dense, rigid supportive connective tissue (tendons, ligaments, cartilage, and bones).

The loose connective tissue, sometimes also referred to as soft tissue, is the connective tissue that is relevant in manual lymph drainage. When we speak of connective tissue in this text, we refer to **soft or loose connective** tissue. This connective tissue joins cells to form tissue groups, tissue groups join to form organs, and organs join to form an organism (▶ **Fig. 3.1**).

Every massage technique that works via the skin to affect the underlying structures involves all the tissues that are present in the subcutis: blood vessels, lymphatics, nerves, and fluids (interstitial fluid). The effect of the massage on the autonomic pathways should not be overlooked.

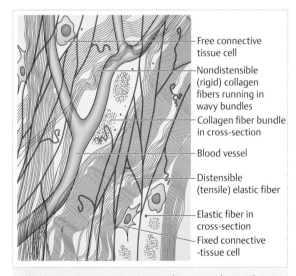

Free connective tissue cell

Nondistensible (rigid) collagen fibers running in wavy bundles

Collagen fiber bundle in cross-section

Blood vessel

Distensible (tensile) elastic fiber

Elastic fiber in cross-section

Fixed connective -tissue cell

Fig. 3.1 Loose connective tissue is the most widespread type of connective tissue. Typical features are the isolated tissue cells and the undulating collagen fibers. Loose connective tissue fills the gaps between other structures; however, it is much more than just a "stopgap."

The connective tissue serves as a supportive connecting structure filling the spaces between all the organs and organ parts in the entire organism. In addition to supporting form, connective tissue surrounds nerves and vessels, stores fluids, and provides flexibility. Since its network contains many defense cells, it also has important functions in the immune system and regenerative processes.

The space between the cells of the connective tissue is filled with **intercellular substance**. Its main components are the matrix, known as ground substance, which is present in large amounts and leads to the cells of the connective tissue being spaced quite far apart, and the fibers. The cells outnumber the fibers. All types of connective-tissue cells are present, though fibrocytes and macrophages predominate.

What is this connective tissue composed of?
- Fixed and mobile cells.
- Collagen fibers, reticular fibers, and elastic fibers.
- Ground substance (interstitial fluid).
- Fatty (adipose) tissue.

3.1.1 Fixed and Mobile Cells

The fixed portion of the cells in the connective tissue consists of fibrocytes and their precursors, fibroblasts. **Fibrblasts** have many irregular cytoplasmic processes that provide their cross-connections. They synthesize procollagens and acid mucopolysaccharides (glycosaminoglycans), the most important components of the ground substance, as well as the enzyme collagenase, which is responsible for the physiological dissimilation (degradation) of collagen.

Fibrocytes are smaller than fibroblasts, less active, and have fewer processes. They synthesize the same substances: collagen, elastin, and polysaccharide–proteins. Connective-tissue cells are capable of producing, in a short period of time, an amount of extracellular substance that considerably exceeds their own weight. To do this, the connective-tissue cell must be supplied with adequate nutrients: energy-rich nutrition plus oxygen. The condition of the connective-tissue cells has consequences in terms of the laws of diffusion, because the extracellular substance (ground substance) to a certain extent constitutes part of the environment of the cells, in the sense of a healthy, "clean" cell environment as opposed to a cell environment filled with disease-causing factors. It does not require much imagination to envisage that cells living in a healthy milieu have better living conditions. Manual lymph drainage "cleanses" the connective tissue through its tissue-draining effect.

The mobile portion of the cells consists of macrophages or mast cells, granulocytes, lymphocytes, and histiocytes. These progeny of leucocytes possess amebic properties that allow them to enter the connective tissue via the blood and move about freely.

> **Note**
>
> *The ability of histiocytes (macrophages) to produce proteolytic enzymes plays an important role in the body's fight against lymphedema.*

3.1.2 Fibers

Because of their structure, **collagen fibers** are a high-tensile, inelastic element (they can only be stretched about 5%), well suited to power transmission. They are found mainly in bones, cartilage, tendons, fascia, and subcutis. In addition, they are also found around elastic fibers, where they have a protective function.

In its stretched state, the **elastic fiber** is as long as the accompanying collagen fiber. In this way, the collagen fiber protects the elastic fiber and prevents it from being torn or overstretched. Elastic fibers, too, are formed by fibroblasts. They always occur as a network, and they are subject to an aging process that reduces their elasticity greatly. If an elastic fiber is stretched for a long period, it takes a long time to return to its original length once the tension has been relieved. This is one reason why, after an edematous extremity has been drained, the skin cannot contract as much as the edema volume has been reduced. Elastic fibers occur in the skin, arteries, lungs, elastic cartilage, and in the connective-tissue capsules of various organs. In the skin, the aging process of the elastic fibers causes wrinkles. In pregnancy stretch marks (striae gravidarum), the elastic fibers have become overstretched and the collagen fiber network has torn. Overstretching of fibers in the lungs can lead to emphysema.

Reticulin fibers have a similar structure to collagen fibers but are much more delicate. They occur in many organs (e.g., liver and kidneys) and in connective tissue, where they form the basic framework. The vascular basement membrane is made of feltlike networks of reticulin fibers.

3.1.3 Ground Substance/Interstitial Fluid

The ground substance is a homogeneous, structureless, colorless, puttylike substance consisting mainly of procollagen, collagen, and glycosaminoglycans (chondroitin sulfate in cartilage, mucoitin sulfate in connective tissue, hyaluronic acid in the synovial fluid, subcutis, and the vitreous body). These substances bind water and other substances. Electrolytes, peptides, amino acids, vitamins, and hormones are also present.

Hyaluronidase is a protein that depolymerizes (breaks down) hyaluronic acid and liquefies the ground substance.

Usually, both hyaluronic acid and hyaluronidase are present in equal amounts in the organism. This balance guarantees a healthy relation between breakdown and synthesis. Adding hyaluronidase would disturb this balance.

Interstitial fluid serves as the environment for molecules carrying nutrients from blood capillaries to cells and metabolic waste from cells back to capillaries. We call it the "transit stretch." This fluid contains many immunoglobulins that are important for defense against infections.

The ground substance consists largely of water. It is movable and of varying viscosity. One might say that ground substance has thixotropic properties.

Thixotropy is the property to liquefy and become a sol through mechanical impact and then revert to gel again. This means that if shear force or pressure is exerted on this tissue, its viscosity decreases toward that of a sol. When the shear force or pressure subsides, the viscosity increases again. The substance is gel-like but liquefies when shaken. An everyday life example is ketchup. It is easy to see that transporting substances through the interstitium is easier when it is in the energy-rich, thin sol state. Shear forces and deforming energies, which must be adapted to the structures of the connective tissue, cause ground substance to liquefy, which one might compare to the liquefaction of synovial fluid during movement of a joint. Heat, too, can dissolve the aggregation of macromolecules in the ground substance, which shows itself in the gel state. Under the sudden application of pressure, connective tissue can display a glass-hard consistency with a corresponding ten ency to tear—that is, the macromolecules have no time to orient themselves in space. Tendon and muscle tears occur during athletic activities not preceded by a warm-up. A typical Achilles tendon tear takes place when the tendon is put under stress in cold conditions. Tendon and muscle tears occur particularly often under sudden, unexpected, forceful impact.

Pischinger (2009) interprets the "cell–milieu system" as a functional unit. Today we speak of microcirculation. Pischinger considers the connective tissue an organ, and by this he means the connective tissue is omnipresent, with connective-tissue cells, ground substance, blood capillaries, and initial lymph vessels, leucocytes, monocytes, and cells where the fibers of the autonomic nervous system end. A network of free axons exists in the ground substance, which release neurotransmitters directly into the connective tissue with regulatory effect, meaning that the ground substance, with its physico-chemical and colloid-chemical changes, is connected via the autonomic nervous system with all other areas of the body. Pischinger's system of basic regulation offers an explanation for the long-distance effect of manual lymph drainage, repeatedly observed during therapy.

Blood and lymph vessels, as well as terminal fibers of the autonomic nervous system, are considered part of the connective tissue. Nerves, capillaries, and cells form a triad that is able to trigger regulatory processes in the connective tissue. These regulatory processes relate to the functions and qualities of the connective tissue described later. Manual lymph drainage is a massage technique that is suited to this type of tissue. It helps regulate the composition and function of the connective tissue, because with the special manual lymph drainage techniques, fluids and solutes can be moved about in the connective tissue in any direction, extravascularly.

When deforming forces act upon the connective tissue, for example, gentle vibration or manual lymph drainage—forms of massage that are suited to the connective-tissue structures in terms of pressure and skin displacement—the connective tissue can be freed of substances that are having an irritant or disease-sustaining effect.

Stimulation of lymphangiomotoricity through manual lymph drainage leads more easily to increased removal of macromolecular substances and water in a sol environment. The connective tissue is rid of metabolic waste, with all the positive consequences for regular cell nutrition and waste removal.

Manual lymph drainage has the following effects on connective tissue:
- The special technique of manual lymph drainage together with the fact that each treatment session is quite long means that the gel state of the interstitial fluid changes into a sol state.
- Through stimulation of lymphangiomotoricity, water and macromolecular substances (the entire lymph-obligatory load and toxins) are removed from the connective tissue.
- The connective tissue is "normalized." **Q 22**

We would like to quote Prof. Weissleder: "It must be assumed that micro-edemas in the connective tissue are the cause of a multitude of diseases." Therefore, by removing the microedema we help the connective tissue to regenerate and reassume its great variety of tasks.

3.1.4 Function and Qualities

The connective tissue is an organ and possesses a multitude of functions and qualities. It maintains the unconscious and undifferentiated vital functions. Its structure is crucial for the functioning of the body because all the information and substances traveling to and from a cell always pass through the connective tissue. With its high water content, it provides a hydroculture for cells; they receive minerals, energy carriers, and building materials from it, and return to it the products of aerobic and anaerobic metabolism. Connective-tissue fibers determine the mechanical properties and also act as mechanical barriers against microorganisms. Many cells and substances of the body's defense system are located in the connective tissue, which makes it an important part of the immune system. Nerve cells (nerve fibers) are tasked with undisturbed communication within the organism. Every cell can absorb any nutrient from the tissue fluid in which it is bathed. If a nutrient deficiency occurs in any cell, it can at any time draw any nutrient from the ubiquitous reservoir without delay due to long transport routes.

Some people are of the opinion that connective tissue is merely a passive transit route for the transport of substances from the blood capillaries to the cells and back. Pischinger (2009), however, classifies the connective tissue as an organ. This leads to the concept of the "cell–milieu system," according to which the cells' quality of life depends on their environment. That seems plausible, particularly as terminal nerve fibers of the autonomic nervous system are present in the connective tissue.

Another quality of the connective tissue is its ability to regenerate itself. When organ tissue perishes or volume loss occurs in the tissue, fibroblasts multiply and fill the defect with cells, fibers, and ground substance. Blood capillaries can regenerate as well. The connective tissue is also responsible for scar formation (fibroblasts).

3.1.5 Adipose Tissue

Adipose or fatty tissue, which provides almost the entire energy supply for the body, is a special form of reticular connective tissue. Each cell stores fat as a single droplet. If the energy supply is increased, the fat droplets in the cells swell and may push nucleus and cytoplasm to the cell membrane (▶ **Fig. 3.2**).

Fat cells are fixed in their environment by elastic and collagen fibers. They can be shifted about under pressure. When the pressure subsides, the tissue returns to its old shape.

We know adipose tissue as cushioning fat in the palms of the hands, soles of the feet, gluteal area, orbit, cheek, and renal bed.

We have storage fat in the subcutis and under the peritoneum of the colon. Excess nutrition is stored as fat that can be metabolized when nutrition is low. The subcutaneous fat layer helps us to maintain a proper body temperature. The interstitial connective tissue can

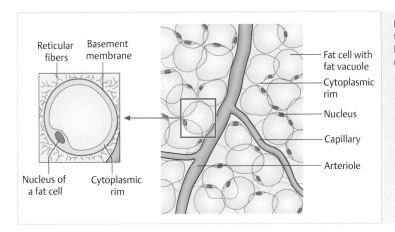

Fig. 3.2 In the adipose tissue, the individual fat cells (adipocytes) are enveloped by a basement membrane and a network of reticular fibers (Faller 2004).

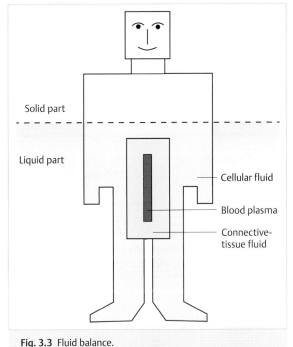

Fig. 3.3 Fluid balance.

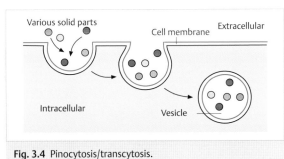

Fig. 3.4 Pinocytosis/transcytosis.

be regarded as a filling between the organs and in the neurovascular compartment. It has a protective effect.

3.1.6 Water Balance

The body consists of two-fifths solid substances and three-fifths a fluid similar to seawater (▶Fig. 3.3)—an indication that all land-dwelling creatures originated in the ocean.

The fluid can be roughly divided as follows:
- Eleven percent (3 L) blood plasma.
- Twenty-six percent (12 L) interstitial or connective-tissue fluid.
- Sixty-two percent (28 L) intracellular fluid.

The fluids are of great importance because substances can only be transported in the liquid milieu. Health often depends on metabolism (i.e., the circulation of substances), which makes it a transport issue.

3.1.7 Protein Circulation: Active Transport Mechanism

In this context, macromolecular substances are usually protein molecules. If the blood protein concentration in a healthy individual is too high, various mechanisms of the endothelial cells of the blood capillaries will cause the protein to be released into the tissue in order to maintain homeostasis.

When blood is saturated with the right amount of protein, a steady intracellular flow of protein takes place. Small proteins trickle through the large pores of the capillary walls and enter the connective tissue.

The active, energy-requiring transport of fluids and solid substances through the endothelial cell is called **pinocytosis/transcytosis** (▶Fig. 3.4, Q 6). This active transport of protein and other substances through the endothelial cells takes place in transport vesicles. In a process called **endocytosis**, the vesicle takes a protein molecule, for example. On the opposite side of the cell, it releases it (**exocytosis**). These vesicles are often found in large numbers in the endothelial cells of venules.

The transport process is as follows: the endothelial cell membrane forms an invagination (pocket) into which it receives a protein molecule from the lumen of a blood vessel, then the pocket closes off to form a small sac (the vesicle). Like an elevator, the vesicle transports the protein through the cell, opens up when it reaches the other side, and releases the protein. Through this transport process, proteins are constantly being transported from the blood into the tissue and back from the tissue into the blood. Other substances undergo the same process. Active transport mechanisms require energy. This also applies to phagocytosis. **Q 37**

A protein passing through an endothelial cell inside a vesicle keeps its molecular structure unchanged, whereas a protein entering the intracellular space directly and crossing the endothelial cell plasma will usually undergo a change to its molecular structure.

According to Földi (2005), all protein molecules leave the bloodstream within 24 to 48 hours, enter the connective tissue, and most of them are returned to the bloodstream via the lymphatic vascular system, so the term **"protein circulation"** is justified.

As mentioned earlier, some of the tissue proteins return to the blood. The average diameter of a blood capillary pore is 80 to 90 Å, although there are a few with a diameter of 100 Å. Albumins have a diameter of 70 Å, which means that they can enter the tissue through the larger pores. Gamma globulins are larger than 100 Å. Albumins are transport vehicles. Their cargoes include water, metals, enzymes, vitamins, penicillins, insulin, and hormones. Gamma globulins have defense functions. Amino acids are the building blocks of proteins and also of cells. Beta globulins are carriers of fatlike substances. Altogether, there are more than 100 different proteins in the blood. One refers to the "vehicle" or transport function of the plasma proteins, which carry vital substances to the cells and carry metabolic waste away from them. The many and diverse tasks undertaken by the proteins show that protein circulation is as important as every other circulation in the body. And proteins circulate via the lymphatic vascular system; their circulation is maintained by it.

So the protein circulation needs a properly functioning lymphatic vascular system; otherwise, there will be blockages and build-ups in the connective tissue, that is, the concentration of protein in the tissue will rise. This will lead to reactive chronic inflammation, which in its turn will result in cell proliferation (fibrosis). **Q 6**

Storage of nutrients: In healthy people, the level of all nutrient molecules in the blood increases after a meal containing all food groups. The elevated nutrient level in the blood produces a high diffusion pressure, which pushes the nutrient molecules through the pores of the basement membrane of the blood capillaries into the connective-tissue fluid, and the level of nutrients in the blood returns to normal. The first thing that happens now is that the cells satisfy their own nutritional needs. Nutrient molecules are then stored in the connective tissue:

- Proteins in collagen and the amino group of mucopolysaccharides.
- Glucose in the sugar part of mucopolysaccharides.
- Fat in fat cells.
- Water in the domain of the mucopolysaccharides molecules.

Thus, all nutrients are stored in the connective tissue, each in its storage molecule. The subcutaneous connective tissue of an overfed person thus becomes several centimeters thick. The connective-tissue storage of an overweight person therefore contains not just adipose tissue but also all other nutrients in the proportion in which they were present in the diet that led to being overweight.

All nutrients travel into the connective tissue for storage or nutrition as long as the capillary basement membrane is healthy, pores are open, and transportation pathways through the pores are freely accessible. This causes the overweight person to be overweight but maintains his health, because the increase of storage molecules in the connective tissue does not have a negative effect.

3.2 Physiology of the Exchange Processes between Interstitium and Terminal Vessels

3.2.1 Molecular Motion: Passive Transport Mechanism

An adult consists of approximately 60% water, half of which is stored inside the cells (intracellular fluid). The rest of the water is divided between the blood plasma, interstitium, fluids such as cerebrospinal fluid, synovial fluid, and the body cavities. Interstitial fluid surrounds all the cells in the body. Basically, metabolism can only take place via this fluid.

The **cell membrane** is the border between the intracellular milieu and the extracellular space. However, the cell needs a great variety of substances to survive and fulfill its functions. In addition, it has to be able to selectively release a wide variety of substances. The cell membrane is very well supplied with proteins for these purposes, and also makes use of a number of laws of physics for transport. Transport is divided into active transport and passive transport (▶ **Table 3.1**).

Table 3.1 Transport mechanisms of the body

Passive transport mechanisms	Active transport mechanisms
Diffusion	Primary active transport (transport against a concentration gradient using adenosine triphosphate)
Osmosis	Secondary active transport ("piggyback" transport against a concentration gradient)
Filtration Q 38	Phagocytosis (absorption of cell debris and bacteria; characteristic of defense cells)
	Pinocytosis (formation of transport vesicles)
	Endocytosis (absorption of particles)
	Exocytosis (release of a pinocytosis vesicle)
	Transcytosis (pinocytosis vesicle crossing the cell) Q 34

Passive transport mechanisms follow the laws of physics and chemistry. They do not require energy input. These mechanisms are as follows:

- Diffusion.
- Osmosis.
- Filtration.

All molecules move owing to their inherent thermal energy (Brownian motion). At absolute zero (–273°C or 0°K), all molecular motion ceases. For example, the wood molecules in a tabletop vibrate in place. Molecules in a fluid or gaseous aggregate state move in a straight line until they collide with other molecules of the same type, ricochet, and thereby change their position (like billiard balls). This spontaneous motion of molecules is the basis of diffusion. **Q 38**

Diffusion is the mixing of substances in gases or fluids that takes place on the basis of this molecular motion. Each molecule is constantly moving.

Free diffusion takes place when solutions are not separated by a membrane. If there is a membrane between the solutions that is equally permeable by all the molecules, this is called impeded diffusion.

Most substances in the body move about via diffusion. Supply of nutrients and removal of waste products mostly take place through diffusion. The distance between blood capillary and cell is the diffusion distance, also called the "transit stretch." For good cell maintenance, it needs to be short. A transit stretch of 0.1 mm is only just short enough for adequate maintenance. If it is longer, the cell suffers.

Diffusion is a substance exchange that is independent of energy: in order to speak of diffusion, a concentration gradient is required. Diffusion always strives toward concentration equilibrium; that is, the movement of molecules is always in the direction of the lower concentration.

For example, the molecules of a dissolving sugar cube at the bottom of a cup of coffee move "chaotically"—they collide and bounce off one another. They begin to move increasingly into the sugar-free area of the coffee, because here there are fewer sugar molecules to collide with. They also move back to where they came from, because they are not moving in a determined direction, but in

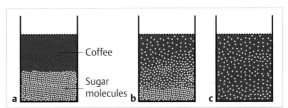

Fig. 3.5 Free diffusion. **(a)** High concentration of sugar molecules at the bottom of the cup, coffee on top. **(b)** Sugar molecules travel into the coffee area (but the majority of sugar molecules are still at the bottom of the cup). **(c)** Complete intermingling. Diffusion is complete; all remaining motion is molecular motion.

whatever direction collisions send them. After some time (4–6 weeks), the sugar would be mixed with the coffee (▶ **Fig. 3.5**). Nobody would sweeten their coffee through diffusion, though: we add energy, that is, stir the cup, and our coffee is sweet immediately.

For the main function of diffusion (cell nourishment and waste removal) to be fulfilled without delay, the diffusion distance has to be very short. Diffusion depends on temperature. The higher the temperature, the faster the molecules move. The smaller the molecules, the faster they can move. The greater the concentration gradient, the faster the particles diffuse. Tissue viscosity also plays a role: the lower it is, the faster the diffusion (▶ **Fig. 3.6**). Q 18

Time is also a factor in diffusion: the shorter the transit stretch, the faster the mixing. The rate of diffusion falls as the square of the distance. If the transit stretch doubles, diffusion takes four times as long; if it triples, the molecule takes nine times as long to reach its destination (i.e., the cell).

The length of the transit stretch is of particular significance for the supply of oxygen to the cells. Oxygen arrives at the periphery bound to hemoglobin in the blood, is "unloaded," and then has to pass along the transit stretch to the cell. There is no way to store oxygen in the interstitial space—every second of our lives, every cell must be supplied with oxygen and carbon dioxide must be removed if cell death is to be avoided. So, the length of the transit stretch is extremely important, and increased length of

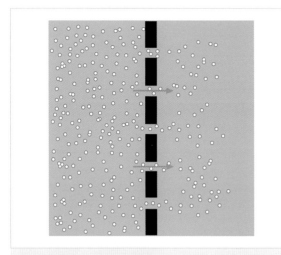

Fig. 3.6 Particles diffuse through a permeable membrane from the side where the concentration is higher to the side where it is lower.

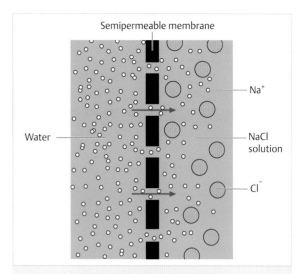

Fig. 3.7 Only small particles can pass through the semipermeable membrane.

the transit stretch can be regarded as "microedema" in the connective tissue. **Q 18**

Osmosis, independent of energy like diffusion, is the name given to the water motion of particles through a semipermeable membrane. This membrane separates the micromolecular solvent into two halves, one half containing few macromolecular substances and one half containing many. The macromolecular substances cannot pass the membrane, but the solvent can. In this case, the micromolecules of the solvent move from the lower concentration of macromolecular substances to the higher concentration of macromolecular substances (▶ **Fig. 3.7**).

In other words, if a membrane separates two solutions of differing concentrations—for example, water on one side and water and salt on the other side—the two solutions have different "water concentrations," because the side containing salt has fewer water molecules. Osmosis strives for concentration equilibrium and water molecules diffuse through the membrane. This causes an increase of water on the "salt" side (= increased pressure = osmotic pressure).

The water-attracting force of salts and sugars is termed osmosis, while **oncosis** or colloid osmosis is the water-attracting force of proteins. **Q 36**

Herpertz writes: "Osmosis is the one-way diffusion of liquids through a semipermeable membrane, in which water in particular moves into the macromolecular solution. The result is a rise in pressure through volume increase in the space containing the macromolecules."

Osmotic force can be measured. Using the previous example, the higher the concentration of salt molecules on one side, the higher the osmotic force. Osmosis is important for the transport of water, salts, carbohydrates, etc., through the cell or capillary walls. **Q 19**

Colloid osmosis relates to proteins. Proteins are macromolecules with a water-attracting force that is called oncotic or colloid osmotic pressure (COP), or suction. **Q 33**

Osmosis can only take effect if there is a semipermeable membrane between the water and the protein solution: for example, the basement membrane of the blood capillaries. The wall of the blood capillaries is impermeable, or nearly so, to proteins. The COP is initiated particularly by the albumins (which are small protein molecules). The protein content of the blood is approximately 7.4%. This represents a COP of 25 mm Hg. This is the force with which water would be sucked out of the interstitium into the capillaries if the interstitium did not contain proteins. But the interstitium does contain protein molecules, which also exert COP, drawing water from the blood capillaries. The difference between these two pressures—in the blood and in the interstitium—results in the suction pressure by which the plasma proteins reabsorb water from the interstitium. ("Pressure" can also be called "suction.") According to latest research results, it requires certain prerequisites for this statement to hold true. **Q 19**

Filtration is a process that takes place along the blood capillaries when a fluid is pressed through the capillary wall owing to the hydrostatic pressure difference between the blood capillaries and the COP of the blood.

The amount of the filtrate depends not only on the structure of the filtration area and the pressure difference but also on the forces counteracting the hydrostatic pressure (COP of the blood). The wave of blood pressure increases the hydrostatic pressure in the blood capillaries so that fluids containing salts and low-molecular-weight nutrients are pressed into the interstitium.

The backflow of interstitial fluid into the blood capillaries is called **reabsorption**. **Q 33**

Since macromolecular substances cannot exit the blood capillaries because of their size, there exists an **active transport mechanism** to take them through the cell, which uses energy (adenosine triphosphate [ATP] dissimilation). **Q 37**

Long-chain fatty acids and macromolecular proteins from nutrients enter the chyle vessels in the same manner (lymph from the intestines is called chyle lymph, or simply chyle).

3.2.2 The Starling Equilibrium

Many years ago, the physiologist Starling stated that equilibrium is present if blood pressure and COP in the blood capillaries are balanced. He observed the forces acting on and in the blood capillaries (blood pressure, tissue pressure, and COP of the plasma and tissue proteins). He called them filtering and reabsorbing forces.

Starling describes four forces:
- Blood capillary pressure is a filtering force.
- Tissue pressure is a reabsorbing force.
- Oncotic or COP of the blood is a reabsorbing force.
- Oncotic or COP of the tissue is a filtering force.

The pressure of the tissue is not a constant. It depends on the elasticity of the tissue, the amount of connective tissue and its components, and the condition of the ground substance (gel vs. sol). The COP of tissue proteins is not constant either.

In Starling's opinion, only the endothelial cells of the blood vessels act as the vascular barrier between vessel lumen and interstitium. This led to the assumption that filtration is allowed by a pressure gradient from inside the vessel toward its outside. Reabsorption takes place when the venous COP (suction) exceeds the blood capillary pressure. It was presumed that 90% of the entire filtrate (100%) is reabsorbed into the blood capillaries and the final 10% are lymph-obligatory load.

Recent findings have called this opinion into question. Present knowledge regarding the transvascular exchange of fluids has expanded and changed. The Starling equilibrium has remained unchanged: equilibrium exists when blood pressure and colloid osmotic blood capillary pressure are balanced. Water does not exit the vessel.

Glycocalyx

New findings show that the colloid concentration in the blood vessel and in the interstitium is approximately the same. These results incorporate glycocalyx (*glykos* is Greek for sugar and *kalyx* is Greek for coat) into the Starling principle. Every healthy vessel is coated with an endothelialglycocalyx, a carbohydrate-enriched coat covering the vascular endothelium. This coat is in a state of constant composition and decomposition, the dynamics of which have not been clarified yet. At the same time, it is serving as a barrier for macromolecules—including proteins traveling outward—and acting as a protective shield between blood plasma and the endothelial cell. This protective shield can easily be damaged through inflammation, atherosclerosis, or ischemia. In such cases, considerable disturbance of the transvascular fluid exchange is to be expected. As a result, an increased amount of substances—mainly plasma proteins—leaves the blood capillaries, allowing the formation of tissue edema. This increases the significance of inflammation even further than previously assumed. The **entire** filtrate can only be removed from the tissue via the lymphatic vessel. Reabsorption into the venous system is reduced to a minimum or does not take place at all. This information is based on the research of Chappell et al (2008).

Under certain conditions, the blood capillaries can reabsorb. This depends on the constellation in the area of the glycocalyx and the COP in the interstitium (high COP at the glycocalyx surface and low COP in the interstitium near the capillaries). Through the reabsorption of water, the COP in the interstitium rises, which reestablishes equilibrium relatively quickly. As mentioned previously, in lymph nodes the lymph can condense, which results in a higher protein concentration in the efferent lymph collectors. **Q 35**

3.3 Function of Lymph Vessels

The lymphatic vascular system is regarded as a safety valve; that is, everything that cannot be drainedvia the venous system becomes lymph obligatory. The lymph volume depends on the structure of the capillary wall and the blood flow through the respective organs. If the blood capillaries are expanded (e.g., to regulate temperature), filtration increases in that area. The same process also takes place during muscular activity. In both cases, more lymph-obligatory load is produced.

As long as the lymphatic vascular system can cope with the additional fluid, everything is all right: the system has a **"functional reserve."** However, once the lymph-obligatory load, particularly the water load, exceeds the transport capacity (TC) of the lymphatic vessel system, edema forms (dynamic insufficiency). Functional reserve (▶**Fig. 3.8**): difference between TC and lymph-obligatory load. **Q51, Q 46**

The quantity of lymph that can be managed by the TC of the lymph vessel in a certain unit of time is known as the **lymph time volume**. **Q 40**

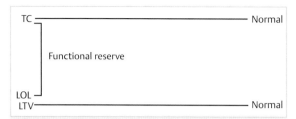

Fig. 3.8 Functional reserve. TC, transport capacity; LOL, lymph-obligatory load; LTV, lymph time volume.

TC is the amount of lymph-obligatory load that the lymphatic vessel system can transport during a certain time unit. **Q 41**

Note

Dynamic edema develops as a result of an increased lymph time volume that exceeds the TC of the healthy lymphatic vascular system (high-volume insufficiency). **Q 51**

There are various causes of this **high-volume insufficiency**:

- **Renal edema**: the body excretes increased amounts of proteins through the kidneys, resulting in decreased COP of the blood.

- **Hunger edema**: the body receives insufficient protein, for example, due to malnutrition or inappropriate diet.

- **Protein-losing enteropathy**: the body excretes proteins via the intestines. The intestinal lymphatic vessels become more permeable, because lymph stagnates in them (lymphatic stasis) or ulcers in the intestinal mucous membrane allow the lymph to flow out. A congenital abnormality of the intestinal lymphatic channels could also be the cause.

- **Vascular hypertrophy**: venous stasis always leads to increased venous capillary pressure and can lead to dynamic edema.

- Cardiac decompensation or right heart failure: **"cardiac edema"** is the result of a very complex process involving a series of neural, hormonal, circulatory, and renal disturbances. The heart muscle is weakened. Congestion in the right cardiac ventricle results, leading to increased pressure in the venous system all the way to the venous capillaries. As a result, venous drainage is impaired; this is known as **passive hyperemia**. It is assumed that the lymph vessels are under a dual burden: they have to deal with the increased fluid volume, while at the same time the absorption of lymph in the venous angle is complicated by the elevated intravascular pressure. **Q 32**

4 Lymphedema

Lymphedema is a swelling of the soft tissue. The underlying problem is mechanical insufficiency of the lymphatic vascular system, that is, the vascular system is damaged or unable to absorb the normal lymph-obligatory load. The result is reduced transport capacity, which leads to congestion of protein in the interstitium. Proteins are macromolecular substances that can only be removed from the interstitium via the lymph vessels. As has been mentioned, proteins (just like salts and sugar) possess water-attracting properties. Proteins that remain in the interstitium attract and hold water molecules. This causes interstitial pressure to rise, which then causes increased filtration. **Q 47**

The classical division of edema was set up by Földi. He divided them into three categories:

- Lymphostatic edema (due to mechanical insufficiency induced by organic or functional changes; low-volume insufficiency, protein rich; ▸**Fig. 4.1**).
- Dynamic edema (due to dynamic insufficiency; high-volume insufficiency, protein poor; ▸**Fig. 4.2**).
- Exhaustion of functional reserve, known as "safety valve insufficiency" (▸**Fig. 4.3** and ▸**Fig. 4.4**).

Additional options for edema classification are as follows:
- Acute/chronic, tending to progress.
- Benign/malignant.
- Primary/secondary.
- According to stages. **Q 27**

In 1892, Winiwarter described the development of lymphedema:

"In the beginning, the skin appears unchanged, just a little taut. Pressing with a finger leaves a depression, but the consistency of the skin and the subcutaneous tissue is more elastic than doughy (as in a simple edema). If one tries to lift a fold of the integument, the skin is noticeably thicker, more resistant, and more tightly connected to the underlying tissue than normal. Later, the consistency becomes increasingly hard and tough; or only part of the extremity remains edematous, while the rest hardens. Gradually, after 5 to 10 years, the circumference of the limb as it continues to swell reaches monstrous dimensions.

Usually, the extremity turns into a shapeless, uniformly thick cylinder, or it narrows suddenly above the ankle as though tied off, like "bloomers," or thick bulges and pendulous lobes hang down past the dorsum of the foot right down to the ground, like the folds of a robe, while the foot itself maintains normal dimensions. If the elephantiasis has spread further distally, the foot turns into a massive, shapeless lump…"

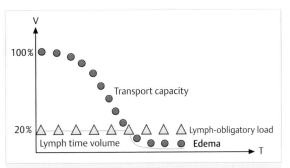

Fig. 4.1 Low-volume insufficiency: the lymphatic system is **diseased** (lowered transport capacity) and unable to process the lymph-obligatory load, the volume of which is normal. This is mechanical insufficiency; lymphostatic lymphedema develops. The transport capacity is decreased. **Q 33**

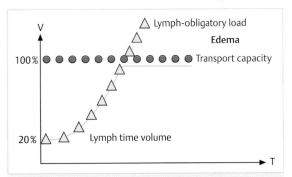

Fig. 4.2 High-volume insufficiency: the lymphatic system is **healthy** but unable to process the lymph-obligatory load, mainly water, the volume of which is **increased.** The transport capacity of the system is exceeded. Dynamic edema develops, not lymphedema. **Q 32**

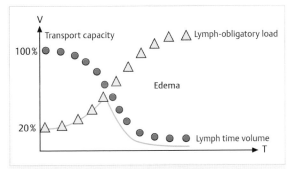

Fig. 4.3 Exhaustion of functional reserve (previously called "safety valve insufficiency"). The lymphatic system is diseased and is unable to process the lymph-obligatory load, the volume of which is increased. The physiological "functional reserve" is exhausted or exceeded. The result is mechanical combined with dynamic insufficiency of the lymphatic vascular system. **Q 33**

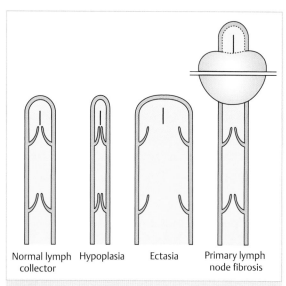

Fig. 4.4 Anatomical causes for a primary lymphedema (according to Herpertz).

Normal lymph collector   Hypoplasia   Ectasia   Primary lymph node fibrosis

Note

*In **lymphostatic or mechanical** lymphedema, the transport capacity of the lymphatic vascular system is reduced and unable to absorb the **normal** lymph-obligatory load (low-volume insufficiency, protein rich).* **Q 33**

*In **dynamic edema**, the transport capacity is maintained at 100%. The vascular system is healthy but unable to process the increased lymph-obligatory load—generally water load—(high-volume insufficiency, protein poor).* **Q 32**

***Exhausted functional reserve (safety valve insufficiency)** indicates that the lymph-obligatory load is increased, as occurs with inflammation or dynamic insufficiency. At the same time, the transport capacity is restricted and is further reduced, for example, by infection in the edematous area. This leads to massive tissue damage and may include necrosis.* **Q 45**

Lymphedema is divided into primary lymphedema (congenital damage) and secondary lymphedema (acquired damage). Both are caused by mechanical insufficiency of the lymphatic vascular system.

4.1 Primary Lymphedema

Primary lymphedema is described as a congenital developmental disorder of the lymphatic vessels and/or the lymph nodes. It is classified into sporadic (95%), hereditary (3%), and accompanying syndromes (2%; Herpertz 2003). The following may be underlying disorders:

- Hypoplasia (fewer lymph collectors).
- Hyperplasia (more collectors, possibly malfunctioning).
- Aplasia (absence of some collectors).
- Genetic.

With regard to lymph nodes, hypoplasia is usually the cause of the disturbance. Characteristic of lymphedema is interstitial enrichment with proteins and water.

Women are more often affected (85%) than men. A congenital transport disorder of the lymph vessels (congenital lymphedema) may exist at birth. It is not necessarily manifested at the time of birth, but may develop later in life, usually during puberty or pregnancy.

Slight injuries (distortion, insect bite) or long air journeys can also cause primary lymphedema, because the lymph vessels that are present are no longer able to transport the increased amount of lymph-obligatory load. In a primary lymphedema, fibrosis forms first at the toes. **Q 55**

4.2 Secondary Lymphedema

Secondary lymphedema is the name given to edema with a known cause. Lymph vessels or lymph nodes may have been damaged or removed by surgery, radiation, or trauma. **Q 33**

The term "malignant lymphedema" is used when the lymphatic pathways are constricted by a tumor or the vessels or lymph nodes are congested by metastases. **Q 53**

Artificial edema is edema caused by the patient himself or herself (self-mutilation). This type of damage is most frequently observed in dermatology. **Q 53**

The various types of lymphedema, their origin, treatment, and relevant precautions are discussed in the advanced therapy courses.

Lymphedema is a chronic disease and must be treated, because it tends to get worse, that is, the volume tends to increase. Collectors degenerate under consistent increased pressure.

The stages of edema are usually differentiated according to their extent:

- **Stage 0:** The absence of clinical swelling does not mean that the lymphatic vascular system is anatomically healthy and functioning properly. This stage may be considered as subclinical lymphedema, latent stage, or stage 0. **Q 30**
- **Stage I:** A visible, soft edema that reduces in size when the extremity is raised. It can reverse spontaneously.
- **Stage II:** Raising the limb no longer improves the edema. Tissue proliferates and becomes fibrotic; often skin changes take place (pachydermia, papillomatosis). It does not reverse spontaneously and treatment is imperative. Fibrosclerotic alterations may already have occurred. The condition is not painful. Stemmer's sign is positive. Skin fold testing is recommended on both sides. With combined decongestive therapy (CDT), volume reduction and softening of the fibrosis are possible. This is the typical clinical picture of lymphedema.

- **Stage III:** This stage is called lymphostatic elephantiasis. It is a more pronounced version of stage II including fibrosis and/or sclerosis that can affect lymph vessels, veins, and arteries and also cause severe skin changes (such as pachydermia, papillomatosis). Reduced immune defense can result in nail and interdigital mycosis (fungal infection). Pain may be present when nerves have been damaged by pressure. Increase in adipose tissue may occur.

Lymphedema is staged on the basis of its pathoanatomical features. A large lymphedema does not necessarily have to be classified as stage III. **Q 30**

Stemmer's sign is measured at the dorsal aspect of the proximal phalanx of the second toe. It is done by trying to lift a skin fold between the thumb and the index finger. A positive Stemmer sign means that the enlarged and hardened skin fold cannot be lifted. Always try on both feet. A negative Stemmer sign does not exclude the existence of a lymphedema. In case of an existing lymphedema, the positive Stemmer sign confirms the condition. **Q 56**

In summary, lymphedema is classified as follows:
- Primary lymphedema can be congenital (sporadic or hereditary) or can accompany Turner's (congenital deformation) or Nonne–Milroy (hereditary, congenital) syndrome
- Secondary lymphedema, in which a distinction is made between benign (e.g., trauma) and malignant (primary tumor, metastases, or tumor recurrence).
- Lymphedema caused by filariasis, an infestation by nematodes that initiates an allergic tissue reaction to filaria antigens, causing alterations of lymph vessels and nodes. **Q27**

The generally known and most effective therapy is CDT, which consists of the following: **Q28**
- Manual lymph drainage.
- Compression therapy/bandages.
- Skin care.
- Respiratory therapy.
- Exercises.

4.3 Possible Complications of Lymphedema

- **Fibrosis:** Increase and cross-linking of collagen fibers caused by fibroblasts. Shift of the interstitial fluid into a gel state.
- **Erysipelas** (infection causing an inflammatory reaction, see later).
- **Lymphocele:** A mass that contains lymph, usually from diseased or injured lymphatic channels, with no endothelial lining.
- **Lymphocyst:** Extension of cutaneous lymph vessels; may also be found along the intestines. The cyst is a cavity with endothelial lining.
- **Lymph fistula:** The cyst can become a fistula, that is, the vessel opens to the surface of the body. The cause is the increased pressure in the lymph vessel. **Q44**
- **Papillomatosis:** Enlargement of the papillary dermis.
- **Pachydermia:** Thickening and hardening of dermis.
- Development of secondary tumors or relapses due to chronic lymphostasis.
- **Nail mycosis or athlete's foot,** because edema is an ideal breeding ground for bacteria and other germs.
- **Malignant secondary tumors:** A person may get a different tumor (also malignant) from the one which caused the edema.

4.3.1 Infection

Infection is the body's (interstitium's) answer to various noxious stimuli. The five cardinal signs of infection are the following:
- Redness.
- Pain.
- Heat.
- Swelling.
- Functional impairment.

The local reaction of the connective tissue causes a local circulatory disturbance with increased vascular permeability for blood plasma and blood cells. The release of epinephrine briefly brings about constriction of the arterioles. The autonomic nervous system relaxes the arteriolar spasm, and local hyperemia and blood stasis follow. The change in permeability is initiated by histamine and serotonin, followed by other biologically active mediators such as kinins, prostaglandins, and others. Granulocytes, macrophages, and lymphocytes move in. Their phagocytic effect determines the course of the infection and whether it will be overcome (▶ **Fig. 4.5**).

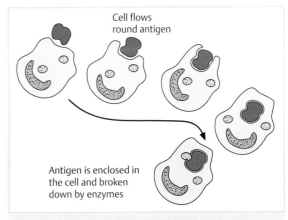

Fig. 4.5 Phagocytosis of an antibody by a defense cell.

> **Note**
>
> **Inflammation:** Epicondylitis (tennis elbow) is an in-flammation without infection.

General reactions to an inflammation can be the following:
- Fever.
- Immune responses.
- Subjective sensations of illness, pain, and exhaustion.

4.4 Physical Reactions to Lymphedema

Interruption of the lymph flow results in stasis and backup of lymph, because the lymph-obligatory load cannot be removed. Lymph vessels distal to the disturbance dilate, the internal pressure rises, and collateral vessels or anastomoses to a different drainage area may open up. Formation of new lymph vessels is also possible (▶ **Fig. 4.6**).

The pulsations of the lymph vessels close to the blockage increase because of the increased lymph-obligatory load. The lymph time volume rises and the transport capacity is utilized in full.

A lymph vessel lying distal to the blockage may grow into another lymph vessel.

Due to the increased tissue pressure in the edematous area, edematous fluid can cross watersheds into other territories via prelymphatic channels, cross-connections between collectors, and anastomoses.

At the cellular level, the body reacts with the migration of macrophages into the area threatened by edema. Macrophages can reduce tissue proteins to small pieces (proteolysis). The fragmented protein cannot form water bonds and is reabsorbed by the blood capillaries. **Q 31**

Except for the last point (the cellular reaction), manual lymph drainage has a positive effect on all the above reactions.

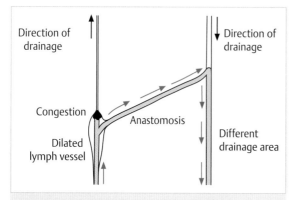

Fig. 4.6 Opening up of an anastomosis into a different drainage area.

4.5 Additional Indications for Manual Lymph Drainage

4.5.1 Venous Edema of the Leg

Phlebedema

Veins transport the blood back to the heart. They move the blood "uphill." Valves (every 0.5–1 cm) mainly prevent the venous return and at the same time excessive increase of pressure in the veins. Varicose veins indicate valves that do not close properly. The pressure in the veins, mainly in the lower legs, increases. Blood cells are forced into the tissue, which causes a bluish discoloration of the skin. Brownish discoloration indicates hemosiderin deposition. This is a visible sign for venous insufficiency that requires treatment.

Long-term overload of the lymphatic pathways is considered the cause of phlebedema development. Particularly during the second half of the day, the patient suffers stasis and swelling in and of the legs. Once the tissue is chronically indurated, the lymph vessels are damaged. A positive Stemmer sign confirms lymph drainage disorder that leads to edema. This is termed phlebedema.

Chronic Venous Insufficiency (CVI)

CVI is a venous disorder of the lower extremities that is accompanied by microcirculation disturbances and trophic changes in the lower legs and feet.

It develops through increased pressure in the veins of the legs and is advanced by the following factors:
- Phlebothrombosis.
- Lack of counter pressure of the muscles in the lower leg (muscle pump).
- Malfunction of the venous valves.

These changes initiate a vicious cycle that causes further damage to the veins with increased valve insufficiency. CVI is classified into different severity levels:
- Reversible edema: dark blue skin discoloration at the medial and lateral edge of the foot.
- Irreversible edema: hemosiderin deposit, dermatosclerosis, varicose eczema, cyanotic skin color, severe tissue tension, and phlebedema.
- Ulcus cruris.
- Positive family history, age, and lack of exercise are considered risk factors.

Post Thrombotic Syndrome (PTS)

The term PTS summarizes all sequelae of thrombosis in the deep veins of the legs and pelvis. There is either decreased venous drainage in the affected section of the veins or insufficiency of the valve system.

The clinical picture of PTS is diverse. It includes everything from discrete swelling to severe trophic disorders with venous ulcers on the lower leg. The first year following thrombosis is termed initial-stage PTS. This turns subsequently into the diagnosis of a late-stage PTS, which basically persists for life combined with the risk of another thrombosis.

In the patient's health history, acute thrombosis is included. There are also silent courses or thrombosis. They are masked by other causes for swelling, such as posttraumatic causes. The level of severity can be determined through functional and morphologic examination methods. Doppler and duplex sonography are suitable methods. The aim of physical therapy is activation of the muscular venous pump through motion exercises. Manual lymph drainage brings about decongestion.

Behavior patterns of the patient are of great importance:
- No standing up for long periods of time.
- Elevating the legs.
- No wearing of restrictive clothing.
- No hyperthermia.
- Exercises to activate the muscular venous pump.

Phlebedema usually occurs in the lower extremities as a result of increased pressure in the venous system caused by insufficiency of the valves. There are different stages: edema, edema with skin changes, and edema with ulcer.

4.5.2 Lipedema

Lipedema is a chronic disease. It is a painful inherited condition that occurs almost exclusively in women. It causes symmetrically painful and disproportional fatty tissue distribution, supported by constitutional factors. In some of the affected individuals, it may result from lipohypertrophy (see Chapter 4.5.3). Lipedema usually extends between the iliac crest and the ankles, where adipose lumps can be palpated. The arms are rarely affected. Increased permeability and fragility of the blood capillaries are known to be associated with lipedema. The small veins and lymph vessels are compressed. There are ectasia and aneurisms of the lymph vessels. Characteristically, the feet and toes (hands and fingers) are usually free of edema.

Women affected by lipedema complain about heaviness of the legs and tightness and fullness of the tissue. They are very sensitive to pressure and touch. The lightest touch may cause a hematoma that lasts for days. The pinch test is positive, that is, painful. It is performed on the lateral aspect of the thigh as a diagnostic test. Ultrasound is used for diagnosis (snow flurries).

There is a marked tendency to edema formation in orthostatism. Weight control from an early age is extremely important. If obesity accompanies the lipedema in the advanced stage, as it frequently does, often secondary lymphedema develops. This is termed **lipo-lymphedema.**

The lipedema can remain unchanged for years if normal weight is consistently maintained.

In true lipedema, Stemmer's sign is always negative. Erysipelas does not occur.

The disease usually begins at puberty, and is characterized by larger hips and heavy lower legs. **Q 54**

The feared "orange peel skin" (cellulite) is diagnosed in stage II of the disease. Compression stockings and compression pants are recommended (compression class II).

Lipedema has nothing to do with obesity and therefore cannot be improved by diet (unless there is an additional adipose component). Normal weight is rarely found. The condition can develop into lipo-phlebedema.

In lipedema, different forms of distribution can be seen:
- Leg: entire leg, upper leg, lower leg.
- Arm: entire arm, upper arm, lower arm.

The edema begins proximal to the malleoli or the wrist with a visible or palpable adipose tissue barrier. **Q 54**

4.5.3 Lipohypertrophy

Lipohypertrophy is also diagnosed as disorder of fatty tissue distribution, with disproportionate swelling of the legs in relation to the trunk. Unlike in lipedema, the swollen tissue is not painful or sensitive to pressure. There is also no tendency to edema formation in orthostatism.

Lipodystrophy is a loss of adipose tissue that occurs, for example, in persons with diabetes.

Obesity, which is related to nutrition, should be regarded quite separately from all other conditions. The excess weight is evenly distributed on the trunk and the extremities. Through a change of lifestyle and dietary habits, the excess weight can be reduced to normal weight. Manual lymph drainage can be helpful to support skin regeneration.

4.5.4 Cardiac Edema

This edema is always of symmetrical appearance and begins usually at the lower legs and feet. It may spread across the entire legs and torso, due to right heart failure based on increased venous pressure with increased filtration and invariable reabsorption.

Diuretics or digitalis are used for basic therapy. In this type of venous edema, manual lymph drainage and compression therapy may also be applied. However, compression pressure must be very low.

If the cardiac edema has not been sufficiently treated with medication, manual lymph drainage and compression therapy are absolutely contraindicated. Overspeeding reabsorption could cause edema of the lungs because of a bottle neck at the venous angle. **Q 29**

Questions

1. Describe the anatomy of the initial lymph vessels. **Q 1, Q 2**
2. Describe the function of the initial lymph vessels. **Q 1, Q 2**
3. Describe the anatomy of the precollectors. **Q 3, Q 4**
4. What are the functions of the precollectors? **Q 3, Q 4**
5. Describe the anatomy of the lymphangions. **Q 5**
6. What is the function of the lymph collectors? **Q 6**
7. Describe the anatomy of the lymph node. **Q 7**
8. What are the functions of the lymph node? **Q 8**
9. What does the term "lymph-obligatory load" signify? **Q 9**
10. What does the lymph-obligatory load consist of? **Q 10**
11. What are the functions of the lymphatic vascular system? **Q 6, Q 8, Q 11**
12. How can lymphangiomotoricity be influenced? What are the inhibiting and sustaining mechanisms?
13. What is prelymph and how is it drained from the brain? **Q 13**
14. Describe the lymphatic drainage pathways of the skin above the navel watershed:
    a) Of the arm. **Q 14a**
    b) Of the thorax. **Q 14b**
    c) The deep lymphatic drainage pathways of the thorax. **Q 14c**
    d) The deep lymphatic drainage pathways of the mammary gland. **Q 14d**
    e) Skin of the head. **Q 14e**
15. Describe the lymphatic drainage pathways of the skin below the navel watershed:
    a) Of the leg. **Q 15a**
    b) Of the abdomen and loin. **Q 15b**
    c) Of the deep lymphatic drainage pathways of the leg. **Q 15c**
    d) Of the deep lymphatic drainage pathways of the abdomen. **Q 15d**
16. Explain the term "watershed." **Q 16**
17. Where are the most important watersheds? **Q 17**
18. What is diffusion? How do temperature, molecule size, and distance affect it? **Q 18**
19. How do you explain osmosis? What is the significance of osmosis for the human body? **Q 19**
20. What are the absolute contraindications for manual lymph drainage and their rationale? **Q 20**
21. What are the relative contraindications for manual lymph drainage and the precautions that may be necessary with regard to treatment? **Q 21**
22. What effects can be achieved through manual lymph drainage? **Q 22**
23. What are the special points that must be observed in the practice of Dr. Vodder's manual lymph drainage? **Q 23**
24. What influences the massage pressure applied during manual lymph drainage? **Q 24**
25. How can protein exit the bloodstream? **Q 25**, pages 21, 22
26. How is protein removed from the tissue? page 22
27. What classifications for lymphedemas do you know? **Q 27**
28. What are the therapeutic elements of CDT? **Q 28**
29. How is cardiac edema treated? **Q 29**
30. What stages of lymphedema do you know? **Q 30**
31. What reactions of the body against impending lymphostasis do you know? **Q 31**
32. Describe dynamic edema and give examples. Why is it called high-volume insufficiency? **Q 32, Q 51**
33. Describe lymphostatic edema (lymphedema) and give examples. Why is it called low-volume or mechanical insufficiency? **Q 33**
34. List dos and don'ts for a patient with lymphedema of the leg. **Q 34** page 111
35. What is the Starling equilibrium? What is glycocalyx? **Q 35**
36. What is the water-attracting force of proteins called? **Q 36**
37. What is the difference between active and passive transport? **Q 37**
38. Which passive transport mechanisms do you know? **Q 38**
39. What is meant by pinocytosis (transcytosis)? pages 21, 23
40. How do you define the term "lymph time volume" (LTV)? **Q 40**
41. What is meant by the "transport capacity" of a lymph vessel? **Q 41**
42. What type of lymphocytes do you know? **Q 42**
43. What are anastomoses? **Q 43**

44. What is the difference between a lymphocele, a lymphocyst, and a lymph fistula? **Q 44**

45. Explain the term "functional reserve of the lymphatic vascular system" (also safety valve insufficiency). **Q 45**

46. What happens in the tissue if the transport capacity of the lymphatic vascular system is exceeded? **Q 46**

47. What happens in the tissue when lymph nodes are surgically removed? **Q 47**

48. What are venous valves and why do veins have valves? **Q 48**

49. What are pluripotent stem cells? **Q 49**

50. List the subgroups of leukocytes. **Q 50**

51. Briefly describe the difference between dynamic edema and lymphostatic edema. **Q 32, Q 33, Q 51**

52. Explain the anatomical difference between arteries and veins. **Q 48, Q 52**

53. What is a malignant lymphedema? What is an artificial lymphedema? **Q 53**

54. How do you recognize a lipedema? **Q 54**

55. Where does fibrosis start in a primary edema of the leg? **Q 55**

56. What is Stemmer's sign? **Q 56**

Answers

1 The initial lymph vessels are the smallest vessels of the lymphatic vascular system. They have a plexuslike origin in the tissue and a single layer of endothelial cells that partially overlap. The vessel is enveloped by a basement membrane, which is considerably thinner than the one belonging to the blood capillaries. This fiber network and the anchor filaments are connected to fibers of the surrounding tissue. **Q 1**, pages 7, 8.

2 Absorption of the lymph-obligatory load from the tissue due to the suction effect exerted by deeper-situated collectors, pressure changes in the interstitium, and osmotic processes. It can also be an active process of the endothelial cell. After entering the initial lymph vessels, the lymph-obligatory load is called lymph. **Q 2** Pages 7, 8.

3 Precollectors have rudimentary flaps, and a few muscle cells are found. They can absorb a small amount of lymph-obligatory load. They are called transport and collector vessels. **Q 3** page 8, **Q 4** page 8.

4 Precollectors connect the initial lymph vessels with the lymph collectors. **Q 3** page 8, **Q 4** page 8.

5 A lymph collector consists of many lymphangions or segments that form a functional unit. Like blood vessels, their walls are made of three layers (intima, media, and adventitia). The middle layer (tunica media) contains bundles of smooth muscle cells. Muscle-free flaps are located proximally and distally in a lymphangion. They control the direction of the lymph flow. The triggering factors for contraction of an angion are: (1) increased internal pressure (increased influx of lymph) and (2) active extension of vessels with manual lymph drainage. Assisting mechanisms ("auxiliary pumps") affect the vessel from the outside, increasing the lymphangiomotoricity. They include contraction of the skeletal muscles, pulsation of blood vessels, increased intestinal peristalsis, and pressure change in the thorax during respiration. The angion also has its own pulsation (autonomic motoricity). It is called transport vessel. **Q 5** page 9.

6 To maintain lymph flow, protein circulation, and recirculation of lymphocytes **Q 6** pages 9, 21, 22.

7 Lymph nodes are lymphatic organs. There are about 600–700 in the human body. They have a connective-tissue capsule with some muscle fibers and (incomplete) trabecular divisions. The space in between is filled with a meshwork of reticular cells. In the cortex of the lymph node, primary and secondary follicles are found as well as nonsensitized lymphocytes and lymphocytes that are sensitized through contact with an antigen. The medulla of the lymph node contains many macrophages (nonspecific defense) and plasma cells.
Afferent vessels enter the lymph node on the convex side of the capsule and empty into the sinus (marginal and intermediary). From there, the (generally) protein-rich lymph exits the lymph node at the hilum via the cortical sinus and the efferent vessels (one or two). Blood and neural supply are via the hilum. **Q 7** page 10.

8 Biological filtration of lymph. Up to 50 % concentration (thickening) or diluting of lymph. Activation of the immune system. Storage of nondegradable substances. **Q 8** page 10.

9 Everything that cannot be absorbed by the venous system becomes lymph obligatory. **Q 9** page 7.

10 Protein, water, cells (cell debris), fat (long-chain fatty acids), and foreign substances. **Q 8** page 10; **Q 10** page 7.

11 Absorption of lymph-obligatory load, maintenance of fluid balance, maintenance of protein circulation, recirculation of lymphocytes. **Q 6** pages 9, 21, 22; **Q 8** page 10; **Q 11** pages 3, 38.

12 Inhibiting influences: local anesthetics, excessive external pressure, pain, and stimulus fluctuation, for example, temperature and current.
Sustaining influences: arterial pulsation, muscle contraction, respiration, and manual lymph drainage. Page 9.

13 Prelymph is the lymph-obligatory load before it is absorbed by a lymph vessel. Prelymph in the brain is drained via the cerebrospinal fluid, along the cranial and spinal nerves, and through the Virchow–Robin spaces (intra-adventitial spaces of blood vessels). **Q 13** page 16.

14 a) Arm: **Q 14a** pages 14, 15.
b) Thorax: **Q 14b** page 15.
c) Deep lymphatic drainage pathways in the thorax: **Q 14c** page16.
d) Deep lymphatic drainage pathways of the mammary gland: **Q 14d** page 16.
e) Skin of the head: **Q 14e** page 12.

15 a) Leg: **Q 15a** pages 12, 13.
b) Abdomen and loin: **Q 15b** page 14.
c) Deep lymphatic drainage pathways of the leg: **Q 15c** pages 13, 14.
d) Deep lymphatic drainage pathways of the abdomen: **Q 15d** pages 15, 16.

16 Watersheds are notional lines drawn on the basis of the different directions of lymphatic flow through the collectors. They are interterritorial areas poor in lymph vessels. Under healthy conditions, separation of drainage flow is possible; under pathological conditions, reversion of drainage direction is possible.
Watersheds can be crossed with manual lymph drainage because it is possible to push the lymph from one drainage area to another (carried away by the initial lymph vessels and precollectors). **Q 16** page 12.

17 Horizontal across the navel and the second and third lumbar vertebrae along the clavicle and the scapular spine, and vertical along the midline of the body (anterior and posterior). **Q 17** page 12.

18 Precondition is a concentration gradient. Mixing of substances in gas or liquids due to movement on the molecular level. The higher the temperature, the faster the diffusion. The smaller the molecules, the faster they move. The shorter the distance, the faster the diffusion. Diffusion time increases as the square of the distance (double the distance = four times the duration). **Q 18** page 23.

19 Particles move through a semipermeable membrane that does not allow macromolecular substances to pass. Herpertz talks about "one-way diffusion of fluids through a semipermeable membrane." Osmosis is important for the transport of water, salts, carbohydrates, and amino acids through the cell and the capillary wall. **Q 19** page 24.

20 Untreated malignant diseases, acute inflammations, acute thrombosis, acute phlebitis, and significant cardiac insufficiency. **Q 20** page 39.

21 Hypotonia, thyroid malfunctions, pregnancy, bronchial asthma, chronic inflammation, sequelae of cancer treatment, cardiac insufficiency, area around a nevus, and toothache. **Q 21** pages 39, 40.

22 Manual lymph drainage dilates the lymphangions, which is considered a sympathicolytic reaction. By applying appropriate stretch stimuli, manual lymph drainage increases the pulsation of the angion and lymph transport is accelerated. The suction effect reaches the initial lymph vessels, with increase of lymph formation and decongestion of the tissue.
Manual lymph drainage has a calming effect because it lowers the activity of the sympathetic nervous system, a pain-reducing effect (Gate control), accelerates immune reaction (lymphocytes reach lymph nodes faster, where sensitization takes place), and decongests—normalizes—connective tissue. **Q 22** page 42, 43.

23 The movements are done slowly, monotonously, rhythmically, working with the skin but not working on it (no sliding). The work always begins proximally. No lubricant is used, if possible. The pressure phase is longer than the so-called zero phase (relaxation). The treatment must not cause pain or redness. **Q 23** page 50.

24 Elasticity of the skin, turgor of the tissue, thickness of the subcutis, and, if muscles or tight tissue (tendons) are located beneath the skin, fibrosis, edema, and angle of slope of the fingers (flat or pointed). **Q 24** page 49.

25 Through pinocytosis/transcytosis from the blood into the tissue and back. Transcellular transport through the cell plasma (albumins) involving adenosine triphosphate (ATP). **Q 37** pages 22, 25.

26 Protein is lymph-obligatory load and is removed through the lymph vessels. Migrating macrophages phagocyte the protein. **Q 25** page 22.

27 Acute, chronic, with a tendency for progression, benign/malignant; primary/secondary; artificial, in stages 0–3. **Q 27** pages 28, 29.

28 Skin care, manual lymph drainage, bandage or compression stocking, therapeutic exercises, and respiratory therapy. **Q 28** pages 110, 111.

29 With medication (diuretics). Stasis edema of the legs may be treated with manual lymph drainage and light compressions. If the stasis edema has not been sufficiently treated with medication first, it is an absolutely contraindicated condition. **Q 29** page 31.

30 Latent stage 0 to III lymphostatic elephantiasis. Lymphedema is staged based on its pathoanatomical aspects. **Q 30** pages 28, 29.

31 Formation of new lymph vessels, transport capacity is utilized in full, edematous fluid can cross watersheds into other territories via prelymphatic channels, migration of macrophages. **Q 31** pages 29, 30.

32 Transport capacity is normal. The vascular system is healthy, functions properly, but is unable to process the existing (increased) lymph-obligatory load (mostly water). High-volume insufficiency is not lymphedema; it is just called "edema" low in protein. The lymph time volume exceeds the transport capacity. **Q 32** pages 25, 26, 27, 28.

33 Transport capacity is reduced. It cannot process the regular lymph-obligatory load. Low-volume insufficiency—high in protein. Primary lymphedema: congenital disorder, secondary lymphedema: mechanical disruption of lymph flow due to surgery, trauma, radiation therapy, etc. **Q 33** pages 27, 28, 29.

34 Therapeutic exercises: Nordic walking, bicycling, walking, and going up and down stairs. Do not exaggerate activities or they will produce the opposite of the desired effect. Prior to any therapeutic exercises, the leg must be bandaged or covered with compression stockings. Possibly skin care before starting the exercise. **Q 34** pages 111, 125.

35 If the capillary pressure = the colloid osmotic pressure (suction) in the capillary = Starling's equilibrium.
Hypothesis:
  Capillary pressure: filtration.
  • Colloid osmotic pressure (suction) in the capillary—reabsorption (disputed).
  • Tissue pressure: reabsorption (disputed by latest research).
  • Colloid osmotic pressure (suction) of tissue: filtration.
  • Glycocalyx. Carbohydrate-rich layer on the vascular endothelium, which is constantly synthesized and broken down, serves as safety shield between blood plasma and endothelial cell. **Q 35** page 25.

36 Oncosis or colloid osmotic pressure/suction. **Q 36** page 24.

37 Active transport mechanisms require energy (ATP). Passive transport mechanisms can function without energy input. They follow physical and chemical laws (concentration gradient). **Q 38** page 23.

38 Diffusion, osmosis, and filtration. **Q 38** page 23.

39 Transcytosis (pinocytosis) = vesicle transport through the cell employing energy (ATP), for example, macromolecular plasma proteins. **Q 6** pages 9, 21, 22, **Q 36** page 24.

40 Lymph time volume is the amount of lymph that can pass through a vessel during a certain unit of time. **Q 40** page 26.

41 Transport capacity = the maximum amount of lymph that the system can hold during a certain unit of time. Edema develops if the maximum transport capacity is exceeded. **Q 41** page 26.

42 T-lymphocytes (also called killer cells), T-helper cells, and T-suppressor cells. B lymphocytes: produce antigens after sensitization and turn into plasma cells. **Q 42** page 10.

43 Lympho-lymphatic connections of collectors across watersheds into another territory, also via initial lymph vessels and precollectors. **Q 43** page 17.

44 Lymphocele: collection of lymph in a space that has no endothelial lining.
Lymphocyst: extension of a lymph vessel of the skin with endothelial lining.
Lymph fistula: a cyst can turn into a fistula, that is, the vessel opens onto the body surface. **Q 44** page 29.

45 Transport capacity minus lymph time volume equals the available functional reserve. **Q 45** pages 28.

46 Once the body's own reactions are depleted, dynamic or lymphostatic (mechanical) edema develops, depending on the cause. **Q 46** page 25.

47 Backup of lymph-obligatory load occurs in the area that was drained by the lymph node that was surgically removed. The body activates its possibilities to avoid lymphedema through bypass circuit (anastomoses), formation of new vessels, and macrophages. **Q 47** page 27.

48 Venous valves are folds in the endothelia of a vein. They can be found most frequently in the legs because generally blood must be transported against gravity in this area. They prevent the back flow. **Q 48** page 6.

49 Stem cells can differentiate into various cell or tissue types, depending on the type of stem cell and its manipulation. **Q 49** page 2.

50 Monocytes, lymphocytes, and granulocytes. **Q 50** pages 3, 4.

51 Dynamic edema: increased lymph-obligatory load, mainly water, or lymph time volume exceeds the transport capacity.
Lymphostatic lymphedema: reduced transport capacity cannot process the normal lymph-obligatory load. **Q 51** pages 25, 26.

52 Arteries: their walls consist of three layers—tunica interna (intima) elastic membrane; tunica media (media)—is made of elastic fibers and smooth muscle cells; tunica externa (adventitia)—connective-tissue layer with elastic fibers.
Veins: their walls consist of three layers, lower internal pressure than in an artery of equal size. In many veins, the internal layer (tunica intima) forms the valves. Middle layer (tunica media) is made of smooth muscle cells. Tunica adventitia is a connective-tissue layer (with nerves) that fixates the vein in its surrounding. **Q 48 Q 52** pages 5, 6.

53 Malignant lymphedema: develops if lymphatic pathways/nodes are congested or constricted by a tumor or metastases.
Artificial lymphedema: caused by the patient himself or herself through self-mutilation. **Q 53** page 28.

54 Disproportional impaired fatty tissue distribution that generally affects the legs only (possible to affect arms), always symmetrical. Great sensitivity to pressure, fragility of blood capillaries, tendency to form hematoma, marked tendency to edema formation in orthostatism, feet and hands are usually free of edema. Cannot be improved by diet. **Q 54** page 31.

55 At the toes **Q 55** page 28.

56 Enlarged and indurated skin fold (second toe dorsal aspect) indicates positive Stammer's sign, which is an indication for lymphedema. Negative Stemmer's sign does not exclude lymphedema. Compare to the other side. **Q 56** page 29.

Part II

Manual Lymph Drainage

5 Equilibrium and Balance as the Aim of Massage

5.1 Fluid Equilibrium

All treatments that stimulate blood flow also increase filtration into the tissue. In order to assure fluid balance in the soft tissue, lymph time volume increases. Manual lymph drainage can recreate fluid balance. The intensity of drainage depends on whether there are any drainage problems in the tissue involved. This is easily determined by careful palpation. Soft, loose tissue has a greater tendency to edema formation. Firm, taut tissue deals better with increased blood flow and requires less manual lymph drainage. Manual lymph drainage should be integrated into physical therapy in accordance with these principles. Blood flow is stimulated first, followed by manual lymph drainage to maintain fluid equilibrium. **Q 11**

5.2 Balance in Alternative Healing Methods

All natural healing systems aim to produce a state of balance in the organism. For example, in acupuncture, which comes from Chinese medicine, therapists insert needles into specific points located along energy paths (meridians) with the intention of introducing or releasing energy; that is, they aim to create a situation of balance in the energy paths.

Yoga has its origin in Indian culture. It exercises body and spirit and its movements contain elements of tension and relaxation. Its aim is creating a balance between the body and mind, thus a balanced human being.

Yin and yang, the acid–alkaline balance, and many other examples in nature display this natural interrelation.

When we employ blood flow–stimulating treatments, the balancing procedure is manual lymph drainage to restore fluid equilibrium in the tissue.

6 Indications and Contraindications for Manual Lymph Drainage

6.1 Indications

Manual lymph drainage (MLD) or combined decongestive therapy (CDT) can be employed in the following disorders:
- Lymphedema.
- Phlebedema
- Lipedema.
- Traumatic edema.
- Postsurgical edema.
- Arthropathy.
- Reflex sympathetic dystrophy—Sudeck's atrophy (posttraumatic osteoporosis).
- Rheumatic diseases.

(*These and additional diseases will be discussed in detail in the therapy courses.*)

On the basis of many years of experience, we also employ MLD in many other disorders. We have been prompted to this by our patients' own testimonies and the often visible results, especially since the results are repeatable. Although there are as yet no clinical trials on the success and effects of MLD in these disorders, we would like to pass these experiences on to our students. Perhaps some therapists will feel inspired to initiate such trials and explore these findings in greater depth. The disorders under this heading are the following:
- Cosmetic disorders: acne, rosacea, scars, and striae gravidarum (stretch marks).
- Orthopedic/surgical/trauma-related disorders: whiplash, burns, keloids, arthropathies, and surgery on large joints.
- Gynecological disorders: mastodynia and lactation disorders.
- Neurological disorders: stroke, multiple sclerosis, and Down's syndrome.
- Autonomic imbalance and as health spa treatment: for burnout syndrome/stress, after serious operations or severe illness in older people, for those on a fasting diet, and in children with recurrent infections ("lymphatic children").

6.2 Absolute Contraindications

MLD may not be used in patients with certain disorders.

At the top of this list are **malignant diseases** that have not been treated surgically or with radiation or chemotherapy. According to current teaching opinion, MLD does not evoke metastases or promote the spreading of tumor cells, but no risks should be taken. In some circumstances, however, MLD is used palliatively.

Another absolute contraindication is **acute inflammation**, whether local or systemic, that is, inflammation caused by antigens such as bacteria, viruses, fungi, chemicals, etc. Next on the list are **allergies** caused by pollen, detergents, foods, etc.

In the case of inflammation or allergy, MLD can aggravate the condition because it accelerates the lymph flow. The pathogenic substances form part of the lymph-obligatory load, and lymph drainage would speed up their spread throughout the body via the lymphatic pathways. The pathogens would pass by the lymph nodes without defense cells or antibodies being activated.

Another important contraindication is acute **deep vein thrombosis** of the legs. Patients often have to remain in bed in order to avoid the risk that a thrombus will become detached from the vessel wall and travel as an embolus to, for example, the lungs. This is why MLD cannot be employed in a patient with acute thrombosis.

Cardiac insufficiency is another absolute contraindication for MLD. This contraindication relates to the edematous area, which as a rule means the feet, ankles, and calves. Deep abdominal drainage must also be avoided. **Q 20**

> **Note**
>
> *Absolute contraindications for manual lymph drainage:*
> - *Untreated malignant disease, including tumor recurrence or metastases.*
> - *Acute inflammation.*
> - *Acute allergy.*
> - *Acute thrombosis.*
> - *Acute phlebitis.*
> - *Relevant cardiac insufficiency.* **Q 20**

6.2.1 Relative Contraindications

The conditions in which MLD may be carried out with caution and with certain preconditions are called relative contraindications.

MLD lowers blood pressure, and this may aggravate existing **low blood pressure** or vegetative dystonia. At the start of a treatment series, a full-body treatment should not be given immediately, but should be built up slowly, starting with short treatment times and small treatment areas. The patient should not feel nauseous. Treatment times are then slowly increased.

Thyroid disorder can also be a relative contraindication for MLD. Whatever happens, the patient must experience the treatment of the neck area as pleasant. This may mean omitting the profundus–terminus treatment and performing only the occiput–profundus treatment. The duration of the treatment should be slightly shorter.

Deep abdominal drainage should be avoided during menstruation.

MLD also should not be employed during the first months of **pregnancy** or when there are complications during pregnancy. In uncomplicated pregnancies, MLD can be employed until the very end and is particularly useful and helpful on legs and breasts. On the abdomen, only the skin technique should be applied.

In **bronchial asthma,** the bronchoconstriction attacks are triggered by the parasympathetic nervous system. Due to its sympathicolytic effect, MLD can prompt an attack. Treatment with MLD should therefore be started slowly and during an attack-free interval. Treatment should never continue for more than 45 minutes. Strokes on the sternum are omitted. Patients must always have their inhaler with them.

In patients with a **chronic infection**, MLD treatment also begins with short sessions in order to not trigger an acute reaction. Drainage begins distal to the focus of inflammation. If necessary, one should discuss the best approach with the treating physician.

Lymphedema is a frequent sequela of **cancer treatment** (surgery/radiation). This edema can and must be treated, but only by therapists who have successfully completed the 4-week MLD/CDT training.

In case of cardiac insufficiency, it is possible to relieve the patient through MLD. But the treatment should be short, cover only small areas, and include a light bandage. The patient must have an entirely pleasant experience. At the beginning of the follow-up treatment, the therapist questions the patient about past treatment and its results.

To avoid unnecessary skin irritation, the area around a **nevus** should not be treated.

Toothache has a special position in relation to indications: it may become better or worse with MLD. MLD can relieve an existing toothache caused by a cold or other disorder. The toothache can get worse if a focus of infection is located somewhere in the jaw. Where a tooth is dead, a granuloma can develop, which becomes activated and painful with MLD. If a septic tooth is extracted but the part of jawbone involved was not cleaned out at the same time, persistent osteitis can develop, which can also become painful due to MLD treatment. **Q 21**

7 Effect of Manual Lymph Drainage on the Smooth Muscles of Blood Vessels and Lymphangions

Blood vessels and lymph vessels are innervated by the sympathetic nervous system. With its sympathicolytic effect, manual lymph drainage relaxes these vessels, i.e., vascular spasm is released.

Lymph vessels are anatomically different from blood vessels. Manual lymph drainage dilates lymph vessels through the effect described earlier. At the same time, however, the pulsation rate is increased. The main influence on pulsation is from stretch stimuli, which may originate inside the vessel, through volume (filling), and/or from the outside. Mislin (1984) showed experimentally that stretching lymphangions length- and cross-wise increases their pulsation rate. The skin displacements performed in the special lymph drainage technique developed by Dr. Vodder produce this longitudinal and transverse stretching of the lymph vessels and thus increase the pulsation.

Increased **lymphangiomotoricity** (pulsation of the angions) will always lead to accelerated lymph flow. The function of the lymph vessel is to maintain lymph flow. Lymph transport, according to Hutzschenreuter (1991), is the **transport of lymph** in the lymph collectors through the main lymphatic trunks (e.g., thoracic duct, right intercostal trunk, and left intercostal trunk). Peripherally, lymph transport takes place actively through lymphangion contractions. In the area of the main lymphatic trunks, the transport primarily takes place through pressure changes in the abdomen and thorax (see Chapter 13.4.2).

It must be remembered that the fluid contained in the various vessel system of the body is constantly moving. This movement takes place in the form of circulation within these systems, and outside them—when the fluids pass the boundaries of the vessels—diffusion, osmosis, filtration, and active transport.

Since every fluid-containing space is a continuous system, the fluids can move freely within it. Factors that impede this free circulation are frictional resistance against the bordering cells and internal friction related to the specific properties of the fluids, that is, chiefly their viscosity.

The main features that cause the circulation to occur are as follows:
- Contraction gradients and osmotic gradients.
- Differences in the density of the medium, which depends on the temperature gradients of the individual spaces.
- Mechanical and motor forces, of which the latter are by far the most effective.

If body compartments are so structured and arranged that the mechanical forces can and do evoke regular movement of fluid, circulation systems are present. Usually, the fluid flows through sharply delineated channels, pipes, hoses, or vessels.

If vessels can actively contract, as for example lymph vessels can, they play an important role in fluid transport—in lymph drainage.

Three types of lymph drainage can be distinguished:
- **Extravascular lymph drainage** relates to lymph formation and the extravascular circulation. Lymph is formed from water that enters the interstitium by filtration and diffusion, from various types of protein that enter the interstitium in the same way or by active transport, from macromolecular lipids from the digestive tract, and from nonmigratory cells.
- **Extramural lymph drainage**, i.e., external mechanical effects on the lymph vessel, is based on the stimulation of angiomotoricity through external forces. These include the following:
  - Movements of skeletal muscles and joints.
  - Pulsation of the arteries (which subfascially are always accompanied by veins and lymph vessels).
  - Intestinal peristalsis.
  - Movement of the diaphragm.
  - Correct abdominal breathing that, together with different pressure conditions in the thorax, causes accelerated flow and transport of lymph to the venous angle.
- **Auxiliary lymph drainage**: Manual lymph drainage as an auxiliary mode of lymph drainage supports the physiologic lymph drainage.

Mislin (1973, 1984) said in one of his lectures about the effectiveness of manual lymph drainage: "If manual lymph drainage did not yet exist, it would have to be invented just the way it is practiced now." He described how manual lymph drainage with its own particular techniques stimulates lymphangiomotoricity:

"Physiologic vasomotor lymph drainage is based on the autonomic pulsation of the lymphangion or, rather, chain of lymphangions. Manual lymph drainage has considerable impact on this drainage system. Its process is composed of rhythmically repeating dilatations and contractions of a series of lymphangions working metachronally. This produces a peristaltic contraction wave. This means that the lymphangions are synchronized in their dilatation–contraction frequency and are peristaltically metachronized in the resulting pulsation. Myogenic automation and neural control of vascular activity via synergistically functioning receptors in the vessel walls ensure coordinated lymph transport.

The main physiological stimuli are pressure and temperature stimuli. Intravascular transverse and longitudinal stretch stimuli increase the 'pulse rate' of the lymphangions. Smooth muscle cells, such as are present for example in the vascular wall, exhibit electrical and mechanical reactions when they undergo passive stretching. Muscles of the vascular wall that possess autonomic (i.e., pacemaker) characteristics need to be stretched to a variable degree that depends on how full the vessels are, in order for the regulation of their rhythmical pace making always to be appropriate to the situation. For all these reasons, the technique of manual lymph drainage, which introduces (though in a certain sense inappropriate) tensile stimuli within the physiological range, has the effect of stimulating vasomotor lymph drainage."

This is achieved through the special lymph drainage technique developed by Dr. Vodder. The pumping capacity of the lymph vessels is provided by the sum of the lymphangions. Increasing the intralymphatic pressure leads to an increase in the lymphatic pulse rate. As lymph-obligatory load increases, **lymph time volume** (LTV) increases as well. This means that increased lymph production, for example, through manual lymph drainage, automatically results in accelerated lymph drainage. The lymphangion contraction rate is also temperature dependent, rising when the temperature rises.

7.1 Different Effects of Manual Lymph Drainage

7.1.1 Relaxing, Calming, and Stimulating the Lymph Flow

The sympathetic and parasympathetic nervous systems are part of the autonomic nervous system. The sympathetic nervous system could be called "day nerve" and allows us to be active (if overstimulated, we may be "stressed"). The parasympathetic nervous system is the "night nerve," the antagonist. It allows us to sleep, to relax, and our body can rejuvenate.

The innervation of the lymphatic vascular system is sympathetic. Manual lymph drainage reduces the activities of the sympathetic nervous system, which results in a relaxing and calming effect. The patient becomes drowsy or may even fall asleep during manual lymph drainage treatment.

Hutzschenreuter (1991) showed that manual lymph drainage reduces sympatheticotonia. The pressure that is applied during manual lymph drainage changes the receptor potential of the mechanoreceptors in the skin. Through the vegetative regulatory circuit, the central nervous system receives the information to reduce sympatheticotonia of the lymph vessels. As a result, the lymph collectors expand. This leads to increased pressure in the lymph collectors, which causes—as previously described—elevated contraction rate of the lymphangions. It can be considered a **sympathicolytic** reaction if lymph collectors expand during manual lymph drainage. In order to achieve this alteration, it is important that the manual lymph drainage techniques are performed with steady pressure increase and decrease, with the exact pressure (excessive pressure causes histamine release in the tissue resulting in hyperemia and/or pain sensation), and a steady rhythm. Treatment of neck, face, and abdomen achieves the best sympathicolytic effect. It could be said that sympathicolysis is equal to indirect stimulation of the parasympathetic nervous system. The flow rate in blood and lymph vessels also increases. But this is a centrally controlled sympathicolytic response. Comparative measurements of the flow rate in blood vessels confirmed the sympathicolytic reaction initiated by the central nervous system as a result of manual lymph drainage treatment (Hutzschenreuter et al. 1991).

7.1.2 Pain Relieving

The perception of pain is termed nociception. The receptors responsible for this process are called nociceptors. They are free nerve endings of sensor neurons of the spinal cord and can be found in all tissues susceptible to pain. Depending on their location, nociceptors trigger different types of pain. There is surface pain, which is perceived by nociceptors located superficially in the skin. The pain can be undoubtedly allocated to the affected tissue. Depending on the location of the nociceptors, deep tissue pain is categorized as muscle pain and bone pain.

Manual lymph drainage has not only a relaxing and calming effect but also a pain-relieving effect. The following deliberations are intended to explain the analgesic effect of manual lymph drainage. As long as pain acts on our skin/body, nociceptors of the skin and body send action potentials via excitatory synapses of the spinal cord through the brain stem to the cerebrum. In the cerebrum, pain is finally perceived as such. We become aware of it and can do something to remove the pain-producing stimulus or treat an injury. As long as the pain continues, nociceptors send action potentials according to the intensity of the pain. Nociceptors are proportional sensors, that is, the greater the stimulus intensity, the more action potentials, and the greater the pain.

We have a number of different receptors in the skin, for example, for heat, cold, and also touch, the so-called mechanoreceptors. When touched, they send action potentials via the spinal cord through the brain stem to the cerebrum, where we become aware of the touch. The nerve fiber of the mechanoreceptor has a collateral in the spinal cord, which leads to an inhibiting synapse. In the spinal cord, this inhibiting synapse has a connection to the pain control center. Action potentials sent by the inhibiting synapse can eliminate action potentials that are sent by the nociceptors (gate control theory) and this produces a pain-relieving effect. Mechanoreceptors are differential sensors, that is, excitation is equal to action potential only if there are stimulation (touch) changes. The pressure of properly applied manual lymph drainage (stretching and releasing) constantly stimulates the mechanoreceptors. The extent of the pain-relieving effect depends on the precision of the manual lymph drainage treatment (**Fig. 7.1**). Q 22

However, there is a limit to the inhibiting effect of pain control. In cases of great pain, the inhibiting effect of manual lymph drainage is not strong enough. We merely speak of alleviation. Nevertheless, this concept takes effect in painful hematomas or distortions. This pain-relieving effect of manual lymph drainage facilitates relatively quick improvement in acute injuries and post-surgical or posttraumatic conditions.

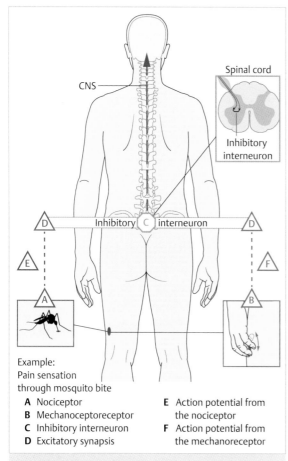

Example:
Pain sensation
through mosquito bite

A	Nociceptor	E	Action potential from
B	Mechanoceptoreceptor		the nociceptor
C	Inhibitory interneuron	F	Action potential from
D	Excitatory synapse		the mechanoreceptor

Fig. 7.1 The gate control theory. CNS, central nervous system.

The decongesting and pain-relieving effects of manual lymph drainage also allow optimal treatment of large extremity edema with tension pains. With the decrease of edema volume, the painful tension is also reduced, which results in improved mobility of the joints. In the joint, lymph is transported through the synovial membrane to the evacuant vessels of the fibrous cartilage of the joint.

The best analgesic results are achieved when we work in the direction of drainage and outside of the painful area, rhythmically, monotonously, and with pressure adapted to the pain. We continue to do so until the affected area can be touched without causing pain. This means we start distally to the pain and work our way proximally closer to the painful area.

Another analgesic effect is due to the decongestion of the connective tissue. The pain mediators located in the tissue (such as bradykinin, prostaglandin, cytokine, etc.) are lymph-obligatory loads that are removed through the lymphatic pathways.

7.1.3 Affecting the Immune System

We speak of an effect on the immune system that has not been proven yet. We know from experience that there is an increase in the body's own defense that can be attributed to an accelerated lymph flow. Pathogens (bacteria, viruses, or other foreign substances) are lymph-obligatory loads and are removed from the tissue only through the lymphatic system. Proper lymph circulation moves antigens quickly to the lymph nodes where they form antibodies that reach their targets swiftly via the blood and lymphatic pathways.

7.1.4 Decongesting: Reducing Edema

Properly performed manual lymph drainage produces an increase in lymphangiomotoricity (pulsation of the lymphangions), which leads to an acceleration of lymph flow (see lymphangiomotoricity, p. 9). The fact that manual lymph drainage treatment always starts proximal to congestions (or edema) is particularly relevant due to its known suction effect on distal lymph vessels (all the way to initial lymph vessels).

Consequently, proper manual lymph drainage treatment can produce effects such as the following:
- Decongesting—through stimulation of lymphangiomotoricity.
- Calming—through relaxation of the sympathetic nervous system.
- Pain reducing—through stimulation of the mechanoreceptors (gate control theory); removal of pain mediators.
- Immunologic—through acceleration of lymph flowing toward the lymph nodes. Q 22

8 Diagnostic Examination and Edema Measurement

Successful treatment results with manual lymph drainage must be documented. In a treatment based on physical examination findings, we can expect successful results in treating lymphedema using combined decongestive therapy (CDT). Ultimately, it is left to the therapist involved to decide how treatment results are documented.

We recommend carrying out an edema evaluation at the first contact with the patient. In our view, this includes the following:

- History.
- Inspection.
- Palpation.
- Edema measurement.
- Body weight and photograph.

History and inspection are performed in alignment with the procedures learned during professional training. Muscular imbalances, faulty posture, and faulty positions are taken into account and are included in the treatment plan if this will be important for successful decongesting therapy.

During **palpation**, fibroses and the softness of the edematous arm or leg and the lymph nodes must be evaluated. The result is documented on an evaluation form. Any other skin changes such as those due to fungal infection, papillomatosis, or the like must be documented as well.

It is particularly important to include skin palpation of the torso. This allows assessment of how far the skin can be lifted off the muscular fascia, and comparing the two sides of the body will give an impression of the difference between the functional and the dysfunctional lymph drainage areas.

The thickness of skin folds can be gauged using a caliper. Different results on each side indicate edema in the affected area of the torso. To compare measurements, they must always be taken at the same location. The therapy team should choose these measuring points with reference to anatomical landmarks, so that the measurements are reproducible.

In practice, the most "economical" and most suitable method is the Kuhnke 4-cm-slice method (▶ **Fig. 8.1**). Measurements must always be taken before the initial treatment and then at regular intervals. Measuring is done weekly during inpatient treatment in a clinic, every 2 weeks during outpatient treatment in the decongesting phase, and once a month during the maintenance phase.

On the arms, reference point 0 is at the ulnar styloid process. From there, measurements are taken every 4 cm as far as the medial axillary fold.

On the legs, reference point 0 is proximal to the malleoli. From there, measurements are taken every 4 cm as far

as an imaginary line between the gluteal fold (posterior) and the groin (anterior).

To calculate the volume of the extremity:

- Determine the circumference of the extremity (in centimeters) at all the reference points (excluding hands and feet).
- Square the circumference of each measurement, and add each result to the next.
- The sum of the added results is divided by π (3.1416). This gives the volume of the extremity in milliliters.
- The unaffected extremity should be measured in the same way to provide a comparative value.
- **Be sure** you always have the same number of measurement points!
- One very expensive way to perform the measurement is to use a Perometer.

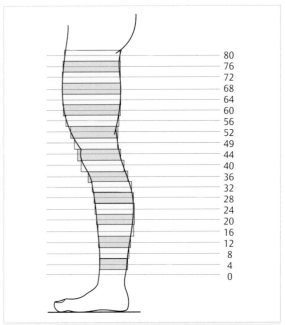

Fig. 8.1 Reference point 0 for measurements is at the level of the malleoli or the ulnar styloid process. Reference point 0 should always be in the same place. Measurement is done from the sole of the foot proximally, and the distance between the sole of the foot proximally and the lateral malleolus in centimeters is noted. In the upper extremities, the reference point 0 should also always be in the same place. The distance from the nail fold of the extended little finger to the ulnar styloid process in centimeters is noted. Measurements are taken on the (lateral) extensor side with the extremity extended and the patient lying down. This ensures a constant reference point 0 for later measurements.

Note

All weight gain aggravates the edema.

Body weight must be checked once a week during phase 1 of CDT. In the maintenance phase of lymphedema, the weight should be recorded at the start of treatment and checked once a month.

Photographs complete the examination and give the observer near-instant information about the outcome of the therapy. Remember to show the same details in each picture, and distance, light, and exposure time should also remain the same. A room without natural light is preferable. Close-ups of fungal infections or ulcers provide an objective measure of treatment progress. The pictures must show the date.

Part III

The Technique of Manual Lymph Drainage

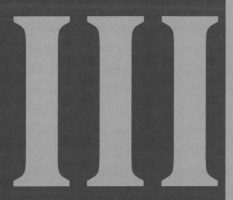

9 Massage Techniques

9.1 The Nature of the Massage

The technique of manual lymph drainage (MLD) developed by Dr. Vodder is a large-surface massage technique that cannot be classified among any of the other existing, well-known massage techniques. A study of MLD will show that the technique is complex and the movements involved require special training. They cannot be learned from a book.

All massage techniques have one thing in common: skin contact is used to stimulate receptors, leading to a particular reaction. Which receptors are stimulated and what effect is achieved are determined by the nature of the skin contact.

To achieve the intended effects with Dr. Vodder's MLD, it must be carried out exactly as taught in its original form at the Dr. Vodder Academy in Walchsee, Austria, and the Dr. Vodder School International, Canada.

MLD consists of five stroke techniques as described later. They can be applied in any combination during treatment. As the descriptions make clear, Dr. Vodder's MLD is made up of a combination of round or oval, small or large, large-area circular motions that move the skin without stroking (or sliding over) it.

9.1.1 Stationary Circle

"Stationary circles" are primarily applied to the neck, the face, and in the treatment of lymph nodes.
- Phalangeal and metacarpophalangeal (MCP) joints are extended; the wrist is rigid and does not move. The circular movement is created through motion of the elbow and shoulder.
- Stationary circles are performed with both hands and in the same direction.
- In the starting position (SP), the fingers or whole hands are placed on the skin in the zero phase. Zero phase means that there is enough tension in the therapist's hands to extend the phalangeal and MCP joints, but the touch remains very light. We call the touch on the skin "... as light as a fly ... a wasp would be too heavy!"
- After the initial contact (SP) with the flat fingers or hand, the skin is moved with a push-pressure motion toward the tips of the fingers and the circle is finished in the direction of lymph flow. The push-pressure movement increases until it reaches the maximum stretching of the skin.
- While finishing the circle, the skin leads the fingers back to the SP, and the push pressure decreases until the SP is reached (zero phase).

9.1.2 Scoop Technique

The scoop technique is used on the extremities. This movement is performed with one hand or two hands alternating. The scoop technique is learned on the forearm:
- The therapist's hand is placed flat on the palmar side. The phalangeal and MCP joints are extended, and the thumb is juxtaposed in opposition to the fingers, similar to a lumbrical grip.
- In this SP, the therapist does not apply pressure, because while in this position the hand is placed in the zero phase with maximal skin contact.
- The ideal push-pressure phase is initiated, still without pressure, by ulnar abduction of the therapist's wrist, "wrist forward."
- The palm is partially lifted off the forearm; only the ulnar side of the hand remains in contact. We say: "Bring the wrist forward, perhaps ever so slightly the elbow as well ...."
- During the following increasing push-pressure phase, with a movement that resembles palmar flexion, we stretch the skin transversely (transverse push) until the majority of the palm is in contact with the skin again.
- Once the palm is in contact with the forearm again, it spirals in the direction of the index finger, performing posterior extension and longitudinal push. In this phase, the therapist swings his or her extended fingers from distal to proximal, not sliding over the skin. The stretch (push) is released without lifting the wrist and the skin allowed to return under the hand. At this point, the movement is repeated.

9.1.3 Pump Technique

The pump technique is used on the extremities. The movement is performed with one hand or two hands, alternating or together.
- The therapist's hand is placed flat in posterior extension on the front of the thigh. The thumb is again in opposition to the fingers. Contact is made without pressure (zero phase) but with the entire hand surface. During the SP, the muscles of the hand are not engaged and no pressure is exerted onto the skin.

- The ideal push-pressure phase is initiated, still without pressure, by palmar flexion of the therapist's wrist. This palmar flexion continues so that the ulnar side of the palm remains in contact with the leg. *Tip:* Make sure that the radius moves forward, not the ulna. In this position, the increasing transverse push takes place with the MCP joint of the thumb on one side and the MCP joints of the fingers on the other until the greatest possible area of contact between the palm and the thigh is reached. The direction of the push is toward the table.
- Maintaining the transverse push, the wrist is lowered until the thenar and hypothenar eminences touch the thigh. With a push-pressure movement, the skin of the front of the thigh is moved proximally (longitudinal push).
- The transverse and longitudinal push phases are performed in one smooth motion.
- This is followed by the phase of decreasing push pressure down to zero, the hand remaining in the greatest possible contact with the skin. During this movement, the skin of the patient returns beneath the hand of the therapist.

9.1.4 Rotary Technique

The rotary technique is used on flat body surfaces such as the back. The rotary technique is always performed with two hands together or alternating:
- The therapist places both hands flat on the back, parallel to the spine. The finger joints and MCP joints are extended. The thumb is abducted in a 90-degree angle to the index finger. The hand lies flat and relaxed on the skin in the zero phase.
- From this SP, the hand moves the skin forward (toward the fingertips) with increasing push-pressure motion and outward (toward the little fingers) in a slightly oval circle. The oval circle is the "rotation" of the rotary technique. This rotation is achieved through slight ulnar abduction and decreases until the zero phase is reached.
- During the zero phase, the hand lies on the skin without exerting pressure and the thumb moves in across the skin toward the index finger.
- Now the palm of the hand is lifted off the skin of the back, but the thumb and tips of the extended fingers maintain contact with the skin of the back. The fingertips slide cranially along the spine without exerting pressure. The thumb remains a fixed point and remains where it was when the wrist was raised. The span of the hand (distance between index finger and thumb) is increasing. Thus, the hand moves cranially.
- Once the angle between index finger and thumb has reached approximately 90 degrees, the hand is placed flat on the back again, the thumb moving slightly medially without exerting pressure. The hand has now

returned to the SP as described earlier and the push phase starts again.

Practice

The fingers are always an extension of the palm of the hand. The work is done not with the palmar aspect of the fingers but with the palm of the hand. This rule applies to the pump technique, scoop technique, and rotary technique.

This technique is also called "moving circles" because during the zero phase, underneath the hand of the therapist the skin slides back into its original position.

9.1.5 Thumb Circles

Thumb circles can be used on all parts of the body except the face and neck. Thumb circles are usually applied with two hands together or alternating. For practice purposes, thumb circles are done on the back of the hand.
- The thumb lies on the back of the hand in the direction of drainage. It is in the zero phase (SP).
- One thumb is moved 90 degrees laterally.
- With increasing transverse push toward the tip of the thumb, the skin of the back of the hand is moved and at the same time spiraled inward proximally. This proximal inward spiraling is the longitudinal push of the thumb circle. The thumb circle is a 90-degree movement performed by the wrist alone.
- During the zero phase, the skin of the back of the hand slides very slightly distally under the thumb.
- Now the wrist moves the thumb back to the SP without exerting pressure, and the movement starts again, this time using the other hand and thumb.

9.2 Duration and Intensity of the Massage

There is no general rule for the **length of treatment**. In many cases, it is stipulated by the patient's health insurance or prescribed by official guidelines (Germany).

The **intensity of treatment** is determined on the basis of the clinical features of the individual case. This requires experience, sensitivity, and intuition on the part of the therapist.

Experience has taught us that the more precisely the strokes are performed, the better the desired effects. The application of pressure can vary greatly and depends on the condition of the tissue. As a general rule, it may be said that the softer the tissue, the lighter the massage pressure should be. **Q 24**

Hastily executed techniques cause vascular spasms and increase the sensation of pressure.

> **Practice**
>
> *Lymphedema is usually treated with greater pressure.*

9.3 Creating the Environment for Optimal Treatment

For the best possible treatment, certain requirements are made of the therapist and the environment:

- Avoid conversations during treatment. The patient is intended to experience your hands. This allows the effects of MLD on the autonomic nervous system to become more noticeable.
- Avoid interruptions during treatment if possible.
- The decision whether to accompany the treatment with music should be left to the patient.
- The room should be well insulated against, or located away from, external noise (telephone, street noise, etc.).
- The massage table should be height adjustable and should not be too soft nor—especially—too hard. The patient must be comfortable. The basics of patient positioning also apply to MLD. Patients with edema of the lower extremities are not given a bolster beneath their knees, but a vein pillow for better venous return.
- The treatment room should be at the right temperature; body parts that are not being treated must be covered.
- The lighting should not be bright enough to dazzle the patient.
- Lubricants (oils) must be used very sparingly so that the MLD techniques can still be performed with precision.

9.4 Treatment Guidelines for Manual Lymph Drainage

The following special treatment guidelines apply to treatment with MLD and differ from the principles of classic massage:

- On the extremities, we always treat the proximal area before the distal area to make room for the fluid flowing in from the distal region. On the torso and head, areas closer to the drainage are stimulated before areas more distant to the drainage.
- We do have a prescribed working pressure, but this is adapted to the tissue pressure in the individual case. Pathological cases may require the use of considerably greater or lesser pressures.
- Each stroke begins with the hand flat on the skin = 0 pressure = zero phase. The increase and decrease in pressure happen smoothly, with the push-pressure phase of a stroke always taking longer than the relaxation phase, which always ends with the zero phase.
- The direction of the push pressure follows the direction of the lymph vessels of the skin. The movements must be performed rhythmically and evenly. The number of repetitions depends on the condition of the tissue and the clinical features of the individual case.
- There should be no reddening of the skin.
- Treatment should not be painful.
- The movements used in Dr. Vodder's MLD make circles with the skin, not on the skin. This means we stretch the skin in the direction of lymph flow without sliding over it.
- Generally, lubricants should not be used. Exceptions might be in patients with damp or hairy skin.
- The therapist's hands should be warm and dry. **Q 23**

10 Treatments of the Individual Parts of the Body

10.1 Treatment of the Neck

> **Practice**
>
> *The therapist stands next to the table, facing the patient. The patient is supine.*

All circular movements of the hand are toward the little finger side.

10.1.1 Effleurage

Five **fan-shaped strokes** with thumbs flat, laterally starting from the sternum. The last stroke is along the clavicle (collarbone), 1 ×.

10.1.2 Profundus to Terminus

Stationary circles from the profundus, middle, along the side of the neck (not shown), to the terminus. Five circles per position, 2 positions on the neck, 1 position in the supraclavicular fossa, "terminus" 3 ×.

Personal Notes

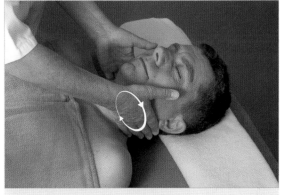

Fig. 10.1 (see Chapter 10.1.2) Neck treatment on the profundus.

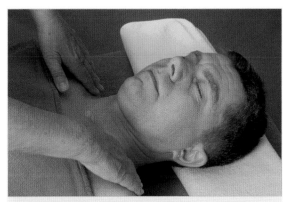

Fig. 10.2 (see Chapter 10.1.2) Starting position for the neck treatment on the terminus.

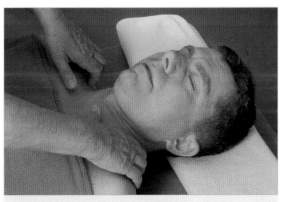

Fig. 10.3 (see Chapter 10.1.2) "Pull phase" during neck treatment on the terminus (bending fingers).

10.1.3 Occiput to Terminus

Stationary circles from the occiput along the middle of the nape to the terminus (not shown). Five circles per position, 2 positions on the back of the neck, 1 position in the supraclavicular fossa, 3 ×.

10.1.4 Tip of the Chin to the Profundus, then to the Terminus

Stationary circles with ring and middle finger beginning below the chin, 3–4 positions, toward the angle of the jaw, from there directly downward, profundus, middle to terminus (see Chapter 10.1.2), 5 circles per position, 3 ×.

Personal Notes

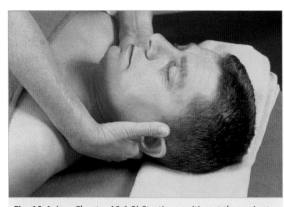

Fig. 10.4 (see Chapter 10.1.3) Starting position at the occiput.

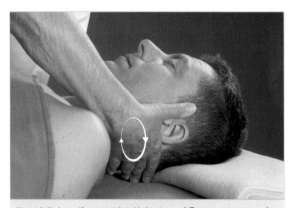

Fig. 10.5 (see Chapter 10.1.3) Occiput: different camera angle.

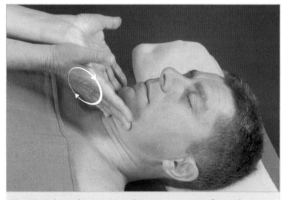

Fig. 10.6 (see Chapter 10.1.4) Starting position for neck treatment on the tip of the chin.

10.1.5 Fork Technique

Stationary circles in a caudal direction, index finger in front of the ear, the other fingers behind it, then drain off profundus, middle to terminus (not shown). Five circles per position, 3 ×.

10.1.6 Shoulder Circles

Stationary circles (not shown) moving the shoulder. Pull caudally and circle medially (toward the index finger).

Then 2 positions on the border of the trapezius, direction of pull and circle is anteriorly and medially toward the terminus. Five circles per position, 3 ×.

10.1.7 Shoulder Circles

Stationary circles (not shown) moving the shoulder. Pull caudally and circle medially. Second position on the acromion with flat fingers. Skin technique. Direction of pull and circle as with the border of the trapezius. Third position is the terminus. Five circles per position, 3 ×.

10.1.8 Profundus to Terminus

See Chapter 10.1.2 (Profundus to Terminus 1 ×).

10.1.9 Final Effleurage

1 ×.

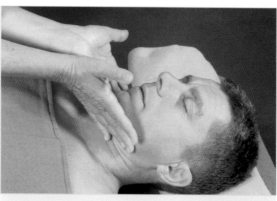

Fig. 10.7 (see Chapter 10.1.4) Midway between the tip of the chin and angle of the jaw.

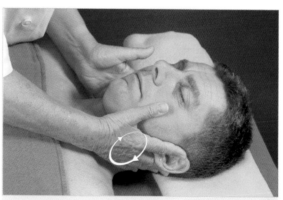

Fig. 10.8 (see Chapter 10.1.5) Treatment of the neck using the fork technique.

Personal Notes

10.2 Treatment of the Face

The therapist stands behind the patient's head. The patient is supine.

10.2.1 Effleurage

Parallel strokes with fingers or thumbs across the lower lip, upper lip, nose and cheeks, forehead, 1 × (not shown).

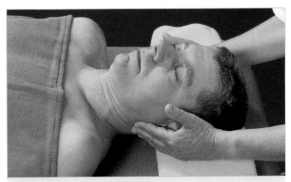

Fig. 10.9 (see Chapter 10.2.2) Treatment of the profundus with flat fingers.

10.2.2 Jaw Area

Stationary circles from the midline of the lower lip to the angle of the jaw (mandibular angle), 3 positions, 5 circles per position, 3 × (not shown).

Stationary circles from the midline of the upper lip to the angle of the jaw, 3 positions, 5 circles per position, 3 × (not shown).

Stationary circles from the profundus down the neck to the terminus. At the terminus, the index finger rests flat on the skin. Five circles per position, 3 ×.

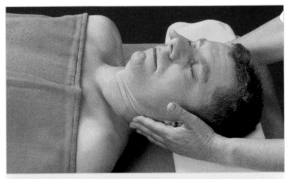

Fig. 10.10 (see Chapter 10.2.2) Midway down the neck with flat fingers.

Personal Notes

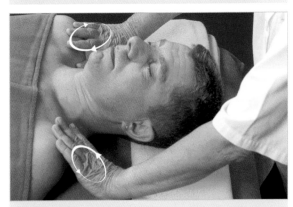

Fig. 10.11 (see Chapter 10.2.2) Terminus with index finger (lateral view).

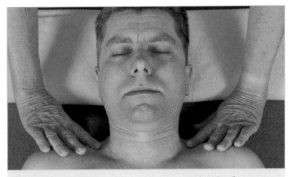

Fig. 10.12 (see Chapter 10.2.2) Terminus with index finger (frontal view).

10.2.3 Nose

Movements on the nose are performed with index or middle finger.

- From **the tip of the nose**, laterally, 3 positions, 5 circles per position, 3 ×.
- From **the middle of the bridge of the nose**, laterally, 3 positions, 5 circles per position, 3 × (not shown).
- From **the root of the nose**, laterally, 3 positions, 5 circles per position, 3 × (not shown).
- **Lateral to the nose**, draining from the root to the nostrils, 3–4 positions, 5 circles per position, 3 × (not shown).

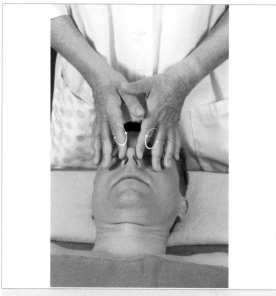

Fig. 10.13 (see Chapter 10.2.2) Treatment of the tip of the nose during treatment of the face, using the index or middle fingers.

Personal Notes

10.2.4 "Long Journey"

Stationary circles begin below the eyes, pass the corners of the mouth, to the tip of the chin, 3 positions, 5 circles per position, direct transition to spiraling 5 circles from below the chin to the angle of the jaw, 3 ×.

Personal Notes

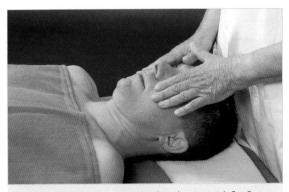

Fig. 10.14 (see Chapter 10.2.4) Below the eyes with flat fingers.

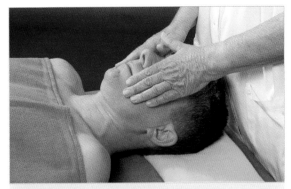

Fig. 10.15 (see Chapter 10.2.4) Corner of the mouth.

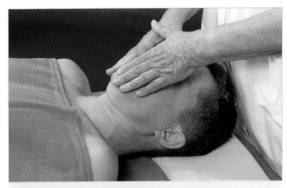

Fig. 10.16 (see Chapter 10.2.4) Tip of the chin.

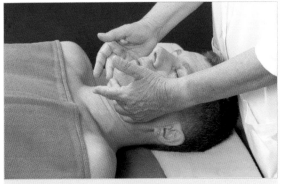

Fig. 10.17 (see Chapter 10.2.4) Starting position for the 5 continuous spirals from below the chin to the angle of the jaw.

10.2.5 Treatment of the Eyes

Stationary circles with half pressure on the tear sacs, using one or two fingers, 3 positions, 5 circles per position, 3 ×.

Pull up both sides with the index fingers, beginning at the root of the nose, 3 × (not shown).

Repeated pressing of the eyebrows on both sides with flat thumbs and index fingers, 5 positions, 3 × (not shown).

Pull up both sides with the thumbs at the root of the nose, circle inward without pressure, and roll out the thumbs over the eyebrows, 3 × (not shown).

10.2.6 Eyebrows

Stationary circles with the index fingers between the eyebrows, then, adding the other fingers, work on at least 2 more positions on the eyebrows without touching the eyeball 5 circles, per position, 3 × (not shown).

10.2.7 Forehead

Stationary circles with flat fingers from the center of the forehead to the temples (temporal bone), 3 positions, 5 circles per position, 3 × (not shown).

Personal Notes

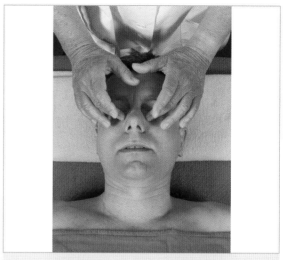

Fig. 10.18 (see Chapter 10.2.5) Tear sacs, position 1.

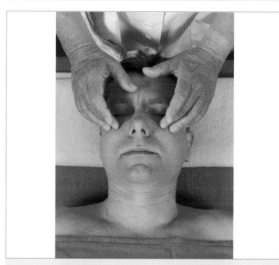

Fig. 10.19 (see Chapter 10.2.5) Tear sacs, position 2.

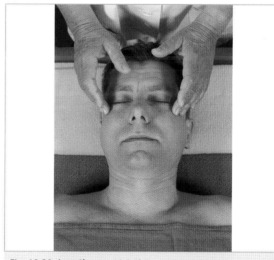

Fig. 10.20 (see Chapter 10.2.5) Tear sacs, position 3.

10.2.8 Temple to Profundus

Stationary circles, 3–4 positions, 5 circles per position, 3 × (not shown).

10.2.9 Profundus to Terminus

Stationary circles, fingers point in the direction of the terminus, 5 circles per position, profundus—middle—terminus, 3 ×.

10.2.10 Effleurage (Not Shown)

Stroke with the ball of the thumb from the center of the forehead to the temples, 1 ×.

   Stroke (same movement) to the temples, then turn the hand inward a quarter of a turn, place the thumb below the eyes, and stroke laterally across the cheeks (lightly), 1 ×.
Place both hands carefully on the face, contacting carefully with the fingertips on the bottom—heel of hands on the top—rest—open the top—open the bottom, part the hands, stroke laterally, 1 ×.

Personal Notes

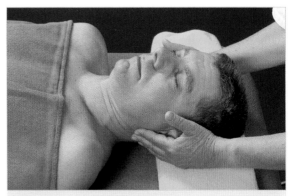

Fig. 10.21 (see Chapter 10.2.9) Profundus with flat fingers.

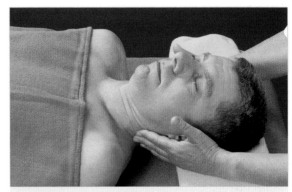

Fig. 10.22 (see Chapter 10.2.9) Midway down the neck with flat fingers.

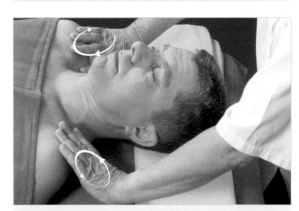

Fig. 10.23 (see Chapter 10.2.9) Terminus with index fingers.

10.3 Treatment of the Arm

The therapist stands next to the patient. The patient is supine.

10.3.1 Effleurage (Not Shown)

Long effleurage of the medial and the lateral aspect of the arm, 1 ×.

10.3.2 Upper Arm

Scoop technique alternating hands on the upper arm. The hand placed on the inside of the arm begins the movement; the hand on the outside lies ahead. Performing alternating movements count to 6, 3 ×.

Stationary circles with flat hands (handwashing motion).

The deltoid is placed between the two hands. Pressure travels from the palm of the hands, across the midhand, into the fingertips, alternating push of the skin toward the fingertips, circling without pressure in direction of the little finger, 3 × (not shown).

Arm lymph nodes, 8 fingers are placed flat on the medial side of the upper arm, fingertips pointing toward the axilla. Stationary circles pushing toward the fingertips, circling in direction of the axilla, 3 positions, 5 circles per position, 3 ×.

Pumps on the lateral side of the upper arm, from the elbow to the deltoid, while lifting the arm slightly, 3 × (not shown).

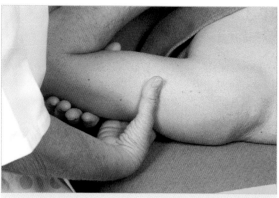

Fig. 10.24 (see Chapter 10.3.2) Alternating scoop technique during left arm treatment. The medial hand begins; the other hand is placed ahead.

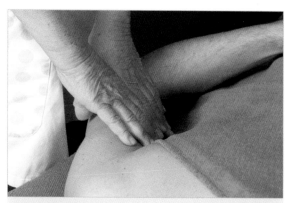

Fig. 10.25 (see Chapter 10.3.2) Stationary circles on the medial aspect of the upper arm during arm treatment (arm lymph nodes).

Personal Notes

10.3.3 Elbow

Thumb circles around the lateral epicondyle, in 2 lines, counting to 5 for each, 3 ×.

Thumb circles spiraling with the same thumb through the crease of the elbow, arm is supinated, from medial to lateral, counting to 5, pushing medially, 3 ×.

10.3.4 Forearm

Scoops on the forearm with one hand, when done, turning the arm from supination to pronation; both sides should be treated an equal number of times, 3 × each (not shown).

Personal Notes

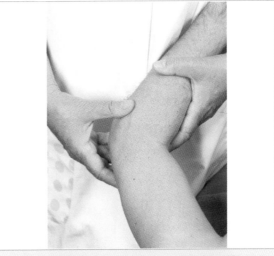

Fig. 10.26 (see Chapter 10.3.3) Thumb circles on the lateral epicondyle, position 1.

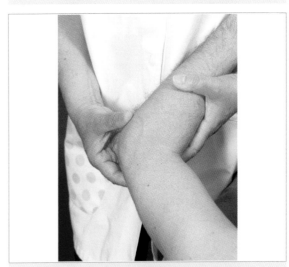

Fig. 10.27 (see Chapter 10.3.3) Position 2.

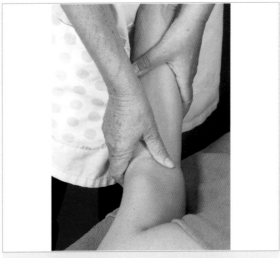

Fig. 10.28 (see Chapter 10.3.3) Spiraling thumb circles in the elbow crease, from medial to lateral.

10.3.5 Hand

Wrist, alternating thumb circles over the posterior surface of the wrist, in 3 lines, counting to 6, 3 × each.

Back of the hand, alternating thumb circles over the back of the hand (beginning on the little finger side), in 3 lines, counting to 6, 3 × each (not shown).

10.3.6 Finger Treatment (Not Shown)

Thumb, 3 thumb circles over the posterior side of the thumb, then pressing the ball of the thumb twice with fingers and ball of the thumb, 3 ×.

Fingers, 2 and 2 fingers, alternating thumb circles over index finger and ring finger, middle finger and little finger, 3 × each.

Palm of the hand, alternating thumb circles counting to 6, then parallel simultaneously counting to 5, 3 × each.

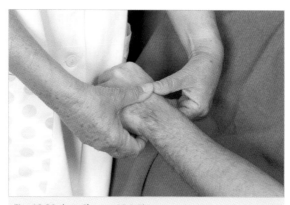

Fig. 10.29 (see Chapter 10.3.5).

10.3.7 Final Effleurage

1 × (not shown).

Personal Notes

10.4 Treatment of the Leg

The therapist stands next to the patient. The patient is supine.

10.4.1 Effleurage

Long effleurage of the entire leg, from distal to proximal, 1 × (not shown).

10.4.2 Thigh

Pump technique alternating on the anterior aspect of the thigh. The distal hand begins, the hand on the lateral side is always placed proximally on the anterior aspect of the thigh, 3 ×. Alternating, count to 6 or 8.

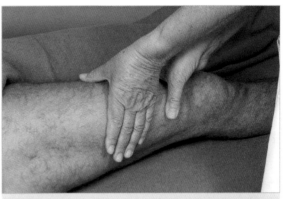

Fig. 10.30 (see Chapter 10.4.2) Alternating pump technique during treatment of the right leg. The distal right hand begins, position 1.

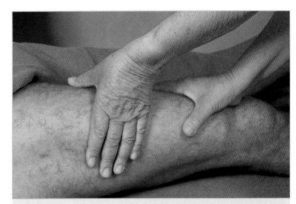

Fig. 10.31 (see Chapter 10.4.2) Position 2.

Personal Notes

Pump-push technique:

Medial aspect: Pumps with inferior hand; alternating superior hand pushes with the fingers, 3 ×.

Anterior aspect: Pumps with inferior hand, alternating with superior hand, using large thumb circles or the rotary technique emphasizing the thumb, 3 ×.

Lateral aspect: Pumps with inferior hand, alternating with superior hand, using large thumb circles or the rotary technique emphasizing the thumb, 3 ×.

Inguinal lymph nodes, fingers are placed flat medial to the adductor canal, 5 stationary circles on 3 positions. The fingertips point diagonally upward, direction of the push is toward the fingertips, circling toward the head, 3 ×.

Connecting the knee, 3 connecting circles—strokes—toward the knee, proximal, applying minimal pressure, 1 ×.

Personal Notes

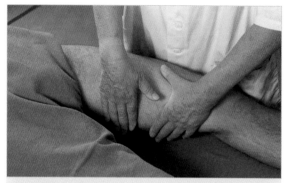

Fig. 10.32 (see Chapter 10.4.2) Pump-push, flat fingers on the medial aspect of the thigh.

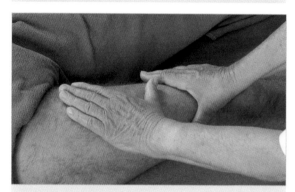

Fig. 10.33 (see Chapter 10.4.2) Pump-push, flat fingers on the anterior aspect of the thigh.

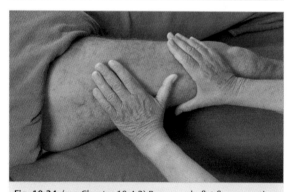

Fig. 10.34 (see Chapter 10.4.2) Pump-push, flat fingers on the lateral aspect of the thigh.

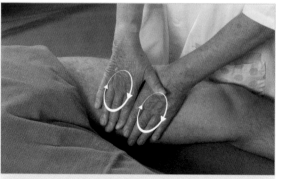

Fig. 10.35 (see Chapter 10.4.2) Stationary circles on the thigh (inguinal lymph nodes).

10.4.3 Knee

Cauliflower: Pump-push. The fingers and thumb of the distal hand grip like flat pliers (lumbrical), without pinching. The push is a thumb circle with the proximal hand. Hands alternate, counting to 6, 3 ×.

Popliteal space: The fingers of both hands are quite flat. The fingertips do not touch. Continuous spirals are applied across the back of the knee, counting to 5, from distal to proximal, 3 × (not shown).

Patella: The thumbs are placed on the border of the patella, 5 continuous thumb circles are performed progressing proximally along the border, 3 × (not shown).

Pump technique: With the inferior hand over the knee, the superior hand supports underneath, counting to 5, 3 × (not shown).

Pes anserinus: Work the pes anserinus (goosefoot) with alternating thumb circles, counting to 6, 3 ×.

Personal Notes

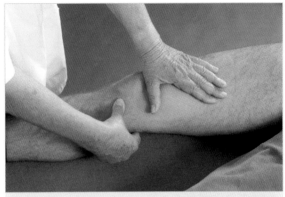

Fig. 10.36 (see Chapter 10.4.3) Pump and push on the "cauliflower" during treatment of the knee, position 1.

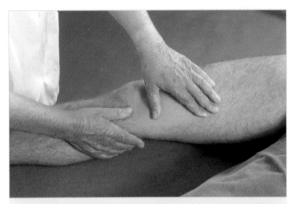

Fig. 10.37 (see Chapter 10.4.3) Position 2.

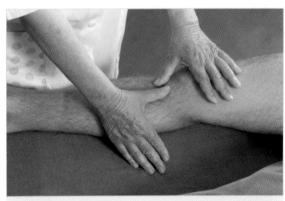

Fig. 10.38 (see Chapter 10.4.3) Alternating thumb circles on the pes anserinus.

10.4.4 Lower Leg

The therapist stands next to the lower leg.

Pump–scoop on the lower leg: Place the foot flat on the table, the knee flexed. The hand on the shin bone pumps, the hand on the calf scoops, counting to 6 or 8. Both thumbs rest on the lateral side of the lower leg, 3 ×.

The therapist stands at the foot.

Alternating scoop technique on the calf, counting to 6 or 8. One thumb is placed on the medial aspect of the lower leg, the other thumb is placed on the lateral aspect of the lower leg, 3 × (not shown).

10.4.5 Foot

Achilles tendon: The leg returns to the extended position. Work with 5 continuous spirals with 4 fingers of each hand proximally. Similar to the technique for the back of the knee, 3 ×.

   Thumb circles alternating, in several lines over the ankle joint, 3 × each (not shown).

   Thumb circles alternating, in several lines over the dorsum of the foot, 3 × each (not shown).

   Lymph sea: Parallel simultaneous thumb circles on the lymph sea; 5 ×, 3 × (not shown).

   Pressing of the transverse arch, 3 × (not shown).

10.4.6 Final Effleurage

1 × (not shown).

Personal Notes

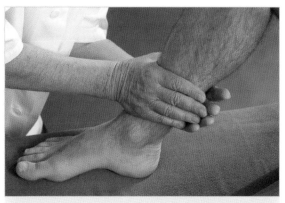

Fig. 10.39 (see Chapter 10.4.4) Starting position for the alternating pumps and scoops during treatment of the right leg; medial view.

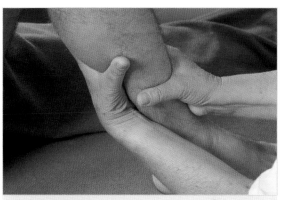

Fig. 10.40 (see Chapter 10.4.4) Lateral view.

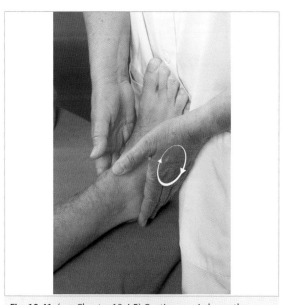

Fig. 10.41 (see Chapter 10.4.5) Continuous circles on the Achilles tendon parallel with two hands.

10.5 Treatment of the Nape of the Neck

Practice

The therapist stands at the patient's left side. The patient is prone.

10.5.1 Effleurage

Rotary technique from the middle of the thoracic vertebrae to the cervical vertebrae, 1 × (not shown).

10.5.2 Profundus to Terminus

Stationary circles from the profundus down the neck to the terminus, 5 circles per position, 3 × (not shown).

10.5.3 Occiput to Terminus

Stationary circles from the occiput down the neck to the terminus, 5 circles per position, 3 ×.

Personal Notes

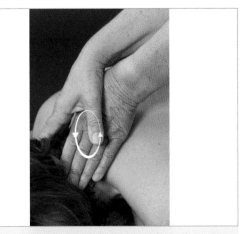

Fig. 10.42 (see Chapter 10.5.3) Stationary circles on the occiput.

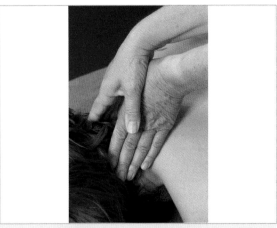

Fig. 10.43 (see Chapter 10.5.3) Stationary circles down the middle of the neck.

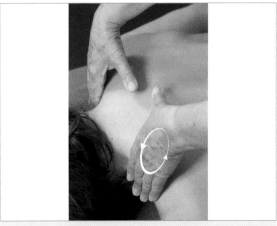

Fig. 10.44 (see Chapter 10.5.3) Stationary circles to the terminus.

10.5.4 Back of the Head

The therapist stands at the patient's head.

Stationary circles along the nuchal line, 3 positions, push toward the body, circle toward the little finger, 3 × (not shown).

Stationary circles in 2 lines on the back of the head, 3 positions per line, then the next line, 3 repetitions per line (not shown).

Stationary circles, on the lateral aspect of the back of the head caudally to the terminus, connecting the end points of each of the previous lines. Depending on the anatomy of the patient (length of the neck, size of the head), 5–6 positions are treated, in terminus supinate hands, 3 ×.

10.5.5 Shoulders

Pump technique from lateral to medial, over the deltoid, counting to 5 (when finished, the thumbs rest in the termini), 3 × (not shown).

10.5.6 "Rabbit" Technique

The therapist stands on the left side of the patient.

Pump technique with the cranial (closest to the head) hand, alternating with pushing toward the terminus, using the thumb and the fingers of the caudal hand, counting to 6, 3 ×.

Personal Notes

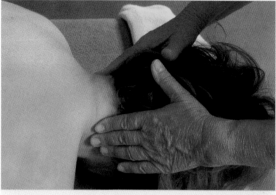

Fig. 10.45 (see Chapter 10.5.4) Lateral stationary circles during neck treatment. Position midway down the neck.

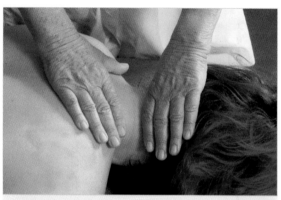

Fig. 10.46 (see Chapter 10.5.6) "Rabbit" technique: starting position, caudal hand.

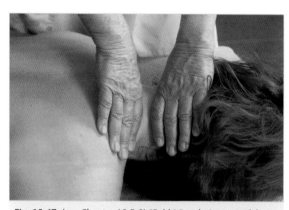

Fig. 10.47 (see Chapter 10.5.6) "Rabbit" technique: caudal hand, push phase.

10.5.7 Skin of the Nape of the Neck

Flat thumb circles with two hands in parallel over the skin of the descending part of the trapezius, paying attention to the cranial horizontal watershed at the level of the scapular spine, 3 × (not shown).

Thumb circles with two hands alternating over the skin of the descending part of the trapezius to the right and to the left, in one or in several lines (in the direction of the terminus), 3 ×.

10.5.8 "Soldiers" Technique

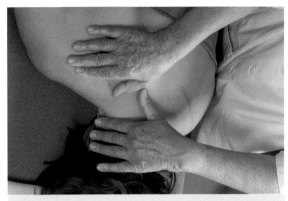

Fig. 10.48 (see Chapter 10.5.7) Alternating thumb circles during neck treatment, to the right terminus.

Stationary circles exerting pressure to the right and the left of the cervical spine with the pads of the 8 fingers ("soldiers"), direction of pressure is down and toward the spine, superior to C7 circle caudally, inferior to C7 circle cranially, 3 × (not shown).

10.5.9 Vibration, Final Effleurage

1 × (not shown).

Personal Notes

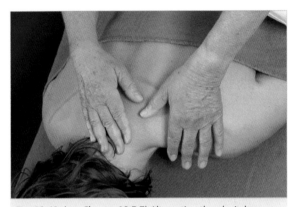

Fig. 10.49 (see Chapter 10.5.7) Alternating thumb circles during neck treatment, to the left terminus.

10.6 Treatment of the Back

The therapist stands on the left side of the patient. The patient is prone.

10.6.1 Effleurage (Not Shown)

Rotary technique in parallel simultaneously, cranially from the shoulder blades, counting to 3; cranially from the middle, counting to 5; cranially from the lumbar area, counting to 7, 1 × each.

10.6.2 Right Side of the Back

Rotary technique alternating over the right side of the back (starting proximally, working caudally and back again, always beginning at the spine, working in lines laterally, counting to 6), 3 × (not shown).

Large stationary circles on the side working toward the axilla (3 positions), push toward the fingertips and circle toward the axilla 3 × (not shown).

Stationary circles on the upper arm, pulling backward and toward the little finger side (2 positions), 3rd position terminus and axilla, direction of push toward the axilla and terminus with flat fingers, 3 × (not shown).

Intercostal spaces: Stationary circles with the pads of the fingers, pressure directed into the thorax from lateral to medial, release medially, 3–4 positions and back again, 3 ×.

The therapist changes to the other side.

Thumb circles alternating on the border of the trapezius, counting to 6, from lateral to medial, the pads of the fingers of the right hand are placed as in a lumbrical grip, 3 × (not shown).

Personal Notes

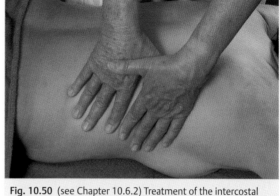

Fig. 10.50 (see Chapter 10.6.2) Treatment of the intercostal spaces, on the right side.

10.6.3 Left Side of the Back

Rotary technique alternating over the left side of the back (always beginning at the spine moving laterally, counting to 6 working in lines toward the side, caudally and back, 3 × (not shown).

Large stationary circles on the side working toward the axilla (3 positions), push toward the fingertips and circle toward the axilla, 3 × (not shown).

Stationary circles on the upper arm, pulling backward and toward the little finger side (2 positions), 3rd position terminus and axilla, direction of push toward the axilla and terminus with flat fingers, 3 × (not shown).

Intercostal spaces: Stationary circles with the fingers, pressure directed into the thorax, releasing medially, from lateral to medial, 3–4 positions and back, 3 ×.

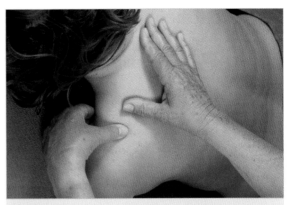

Fig. 10.51 (see Chapter 10.6.3) Thumb circles alternating over the border of the left trapezius during treatment of the back, after changing sides for the second time.

> **Practice**
>
> *The therapist changes to the other side.*

Thumb circles alternating on the border of the trapezius, from lateral to medial, counting to 6, the pads of the fingers of the left hand are placed as in a lumbrical grip, 3 ×.

10.6.4 Extensors of the Spine

Rotary technique along the extensors of the spine, in parallel and alternating—varying the rhythm—several repetitions (not shown).

Personal Notes

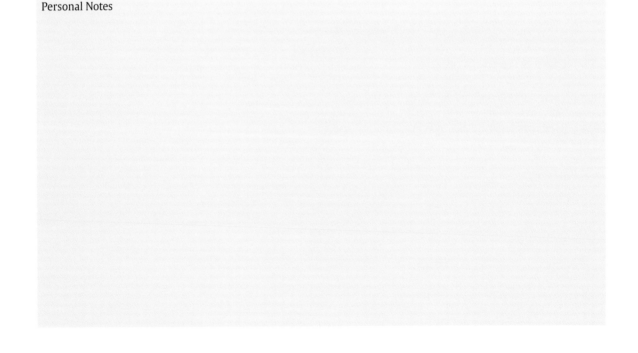

10.6.5 Triangle between the Shoulder Blades

Flat thumb circles in parallel simultaneously between the shoulder blades, counting to 5, 3 ×.

Thumb circles alternating, counting to 6, from the spine to the border of the right shoulder blade in at least 3 lines and to the left shoulder blade in at least 3 lines, 3 × each.

Personal Notes

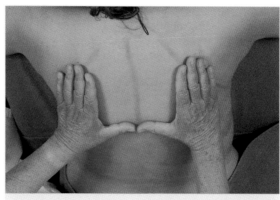

Fig. 10.52 (see Chapter 10.6.5) Treatment of the triangle between the shoulder blades; simultaneous flat thumb circles on each side of the spine.

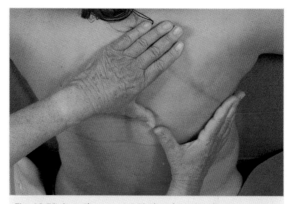

Fig. 10.53 (see Chapter 10.6.5) Thumb circles alternating to the right.

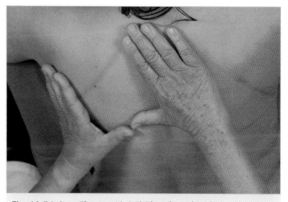

Fig. 10.54 (see Chapter 10.6.5) Thumb circles alternating to the left.

Stationary circles with flat fingers on 2–3 positions between the spine and the border of the shoulder blade, right and left, pushing toward the axilla; on the right, circles to the right; on the left, circles to the left, 3 × each.

10.6.6 "Soldiers" Technique (Not Shown)

Stationary circles with the pads of the 8 fingers to the right and the left of the spine.

The direction of pressure is down (into the table) and toward the spine, circling toward the head. Treat the entire spine, 3 ×.

10.6.7 Vibration and Final Effleurage

1 × (not shown).

Personal Notes

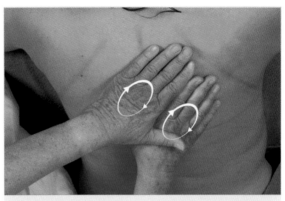

Fig. 10.55 (see Chapter 10.6.5) Stationary circles, in parallel with both hands flat, in the triangle between the shoulder blades toward the right.

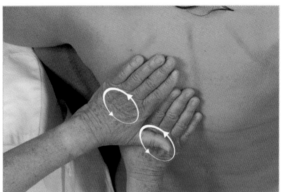

Fig. 10.56 (see Chapter 10.6.5) Stationary circles, in parallel with both hands flat, in the triangle between the shoulder blades toward the left.

10.7 Treatment of the Buttocks

Practice

The therapist stands on the left side of the patient. The patient is prone.

10.7.1 Effleurage

Rotary technique simultaneously, counting to 5, from the sacrum along the lumbar vertebrae, 1 × (not shown).

10.7.2 Right Buttock

Rotary technique alternating, from the lumbar vertebrae and gluteals in several lines to the side and back, counting to 6 each time, 3 × (not shown).

Stationary circles, one hand on top of the other over the iliac crest. Push toward the fingertips and circle without pressure toward the head. Three positions, beginning laterally, moving medially to the spine, and 3 positions back to lateral, 3 ×.

Stationary circles inferior to the iliac crest, several positions on 3 imaginary half circles on the gluteals. Fingers are placed in the direction of the lymph flow, push toward the fingertips, circle toward the feet, 3 × (not shown).

"Soldiers" technique: Stationary circles with the tips of 8 fingers along the sacrum and the lumbar vertebrae, direction of pressure is down (into the table), toward the spine, and circles toward the head, 2 positions, 3 × (not shown).

Stationary circles on the quadratus lumborum between the iliac crest and the 12th rib, prestretching the skin, from lateral to medial, that is, toward the spine, 2–3 positions, 3 × (not shown).

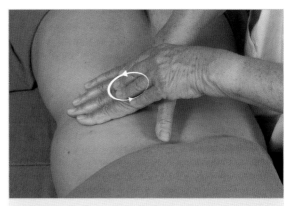

Fig. 10.57 (see Chapter 10.7.2) One hand on top of the other over the iliac crest.

Practice

The therapist changes to the other side.

Personal Notes

10.7.3 Left Buttock

Rotary technique alternating, from the lumbar vertebrae and gluteals in several lines to the side and back, counting to 6 each time, 3 × (not shown).

Stationary circles, one hand on top of the other over the iliac crest. Push toward the fingertips and circle without pressure toward the head. Three positions, beginning laterally, moving medially to the spine, and 3 positions back to lateral, 3 × (not shown).

Stationary circles inferior to the iliac crest, several positions on 3 imaginary half circles on the gluteals radiating from the sacrum, back and forth. Fingers are placed in the direction of the lymph flow, push toward the fingertips, circle toward the feet, 5 circles per position, 3 × (not shown).

"Soldiers" technique: Stationary circles with the tips of 8 fingers along the sacrum and the lumbar vertebrae, direction of pressure is down (into the table), toward the spine, and circles toward the head, 2 positions, 3 × (not shown).

Stationary circles on the quadratus lumborum between the iliac crest and the 12th rib, prestretching the skin, from lateral to medial, that is, toward the spine, 2–3 positions, 3 × (not shown).

10.7.4 Sacral Triangle

Flat, simultaneous thumb circles on the sacral triangle, toward the head, counting to 5, 3 ×.

Alternating thumb circles in at least 3 lines toward the right and toward the left, counting to 6, 3 × each.

Personal Notes

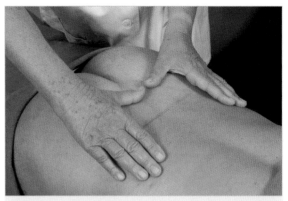

Fig. 10.58 (see Chapter 10.7.4) Simultaneous thumb circles on the sacrum.

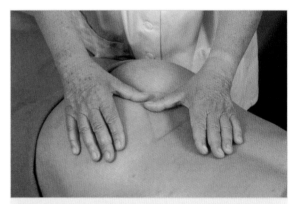

Fig. 10.59 (see Chapter 10.7.4) Alternating thumb circles to the right.

Fig. 10.60 (see Chapter 10.7.4) Alternating thumb circles to the left.

Stationary circles with flat fingers on the sacral triangle, push laterally, circles on the left side toward the left, and circles on the right side toward the right, 3 ×.

10.7.5 Vibration and Final Effleurage

1 × (not shown).

Personal Notes

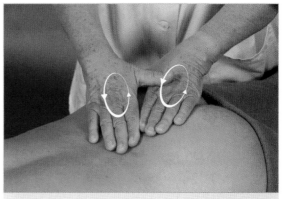

Fig. 10.61 (see Chapter 10.7.4) Stationary circles with flat fingers toward the left on the sacral triangle during treatment of the buttocks.

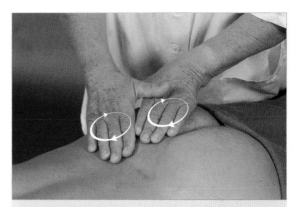

Fig. 10.62 (see Chapter 10.7.4) Stationary circles with flat fingers toward the right.

10.8 Treatment of the Chest

The therapist stands on the right side of the patient. The patient is supine.

10.8.1 Effleurage

Rotary technique emphasizing the thumb, from the sternum to both axillae, parallel movements, counting to 5, 1 × (not shown).

10.8.2 Left Side

Stationary circles with extended flat fingers, lateral part of the breast, 3 × (not shown).

Alternating stationary circles at the same position, counting to 6, 3 × (not shown).

Alternating pump-push across the breast. The caudal hand pumps as far as the nipple and the cranial hand pushes with the rotary technique emphasizing the thumb, toward the axilla, 3 ×.

Thorax (ribcage below the breast): **Alternating rotary technique** across the thorax to the side. The hand closer to the breast begins and works ahead, 3 ×.

Treatment of the intercostal spaces: Stationary circles with spread fingers, pressure directed into the thorax, from lateral to medial and back, 3–4 positions, 3 ×.

Personal Notes

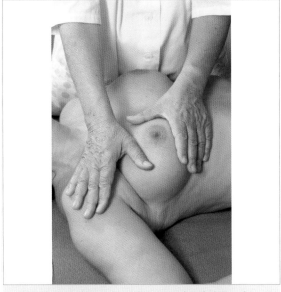

Fig. 10.63 (see Chapter 10.8.3) Pump and push during the treatment of the chest.

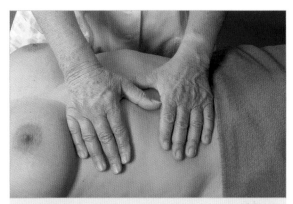

Fig. 10.64 (see Chapter 10.8.3) Alternating rotary technique.

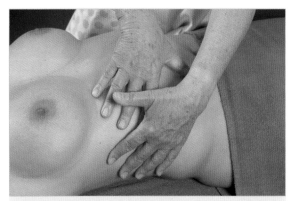

Fig. 10.65 (see Chapter 10.8.3) Treatment of the intercostal spaces.

"Soldiers" technique: On the origin of the ribs at the sternum with 8 fingers. Light pressure into the sternum and circles toward the head, 2–3 positions, 3 ×.

Large stationary circles on several positions with 8 fingers on the side of the chest as far as the axilla. Push toward the fingertips and circle toward the axilla, 3 ×.

10.8.3 Right Side

The same sequences and numbers of repetitions are performed as on the left side.

Stationary circles with extended flat fingers, lateral part of the breast, 3 × (not shown).

Alternating stationary circles at the same position, counting to 6, 3 × (not shown).

Alternating pump-push across the breast. The caudal hand pumps to the nipple and the cranial hand pushes with the rotary technique emphasizing the thumb, toward the axilla, 3 ×.

Thorax: Alternating rotary technique across the thorax to the side. The hand closer to the breast begins and works ahead.

Treatment of the intercostal spaces: Stationary circles with spread fingers, pressure directed into the thorax, from lateral to medial and back, 3–4 positions, 3 ×.

"Soldiers" technique: On the origin of the ribs at the sternum with 8 fingers. Light pressure into the sternum and circles toward the head, 2–3 positions, 3 ×.

Large stationary circles on several positions with 8 fingers on the side of the chest as far as the axilla. Push toward the fingertips and circle toward the axilla, 3 ×.

Personal Notes

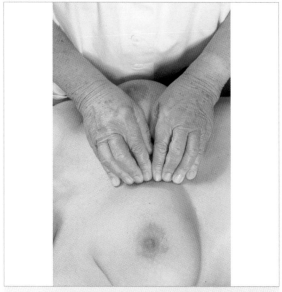

Fig. 10.66 (see Chapter 10.8.3) Treatment of the insertion of the ribs at the sternum.

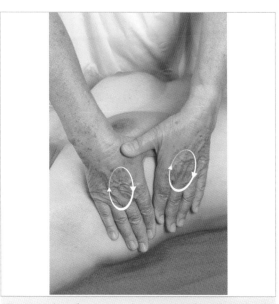

Fig. 10.67 (see Chapter 10.8.3) Stationary circles with two hands simultaneously on the right side during treatment of the chest.

10.8.4 "Seven" Technique

Rotary technique in parallel simultaneously along the costal arches (below the breast) to the sides, counting to 4, then 3 continuous spirals with flat fingers to the axilla, counting to 7, 3 ×.

10.8.5 Final Effleurage

1 × (not shown).

Personal Notes

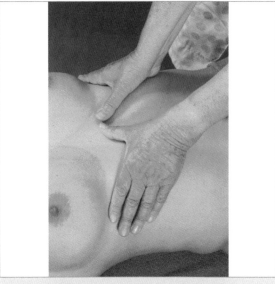

Fig. 10.68 (see Chapter 10.8.4) "Seven" technique during treatment of the chest. Rotary technique.

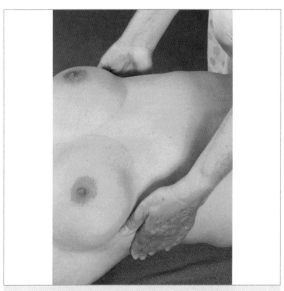

Fig. 10.69 (see Chapter 10.8.4) Stationary circles cranially.

10.9 Treatment of the Abdomen

Manual lymph drainage treatment of the abdomen has a stimulating and regulating effect on the intestinal peristalsis.

10.9.1 Effleurage

Rotary technique from the pubic bone to below the sternum, 1 × (not shown).

10.9.2 Solar Plexus

Strokes over the solar plexus with the flat hand, several repetitions, 5 × (not shown).

10.9.3 Colon Strokes

Strokes along the descending colon (alternating hands), 3 × (not shown).

Strokes in a triangular pattern with both hands along the descending, ascending, and transverse colon, 3 × (not shown).

Personal Notes

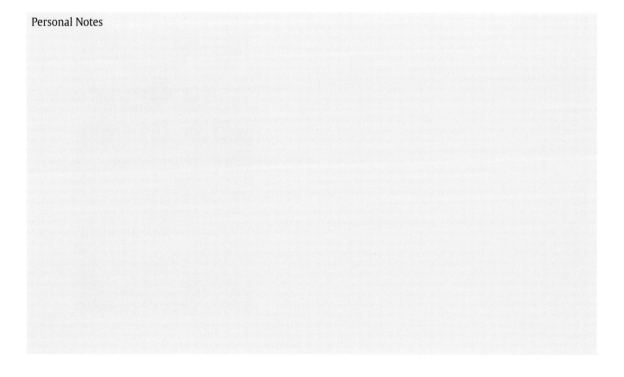

10.9.4 Treatment of the Colon

Stationary circles (one hand on top of the other) along the descending colon (3–4 positions, 5 oval circles per position) emphasizing the direction of the colon during the pull-pressure phase, circling medially each time without pressure. Along the ascending colon (3–4 positions, 5 oval circles per position) push toward the fingertips. Along the transverse colon (5–6 positions, 5 oval circles per position) also push toward the fingertips, 3 ×.

Personal Notes

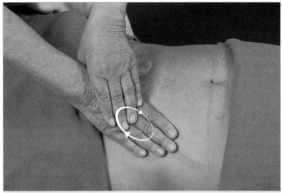

Fig. 10.70 (see Chapter 10.9.4) Treatment of the descending colon.

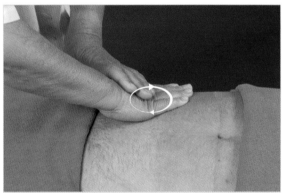

Fig. 10.71 (see Chapter 10.9.4) Treatment of the ascending colon.

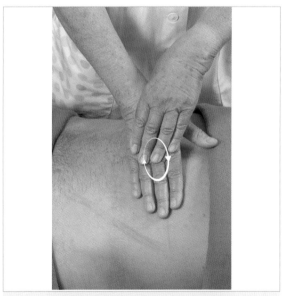

Fig. 10.72 (see Chapter 10.9.4) Treatment of the transverse colon.

10.9.5 Weight Reduction Technique (Treatment of the Small Intestine)

Alternating rotary technique back and forth across the lower abdomen, counting to 6 or 8, staying below the navel if possible, 3 ×.

10.9.6 Treatment of Deep Lymph Vessels/Nodes

Deep stationary circles with fingers placed flat on the lateral aspect of the pubic bone and next to the rectus abdominis. Before the pressure phase, the skin is pushed distally, that is, toward the feet, without pressure. Pressure is then exerted downward (into the table) and toward the cisterna chyli. Keep movements slow and observe the patient (treatment may cause pain), 5 circles on the right and 5 circles on the left side, 3 ×.

10.9.7 Final Effleurage with Breathing

Flat rotary technique from the pubic bone to below the sternum during inspiration; during expiration, parallel strokes with the thumbs along the costal arches, then with the fingers along the iliac crest and the inguinal ligaments to the pubic bone, 1 × (not shown).

Personal Notes

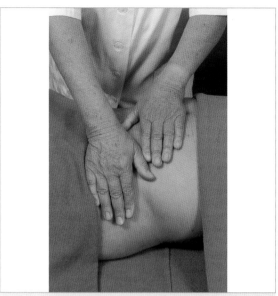

Fig. 10.73 (see Chapter 10.9.5) Weight reduction technique: alternating rotary technique, starting backward.

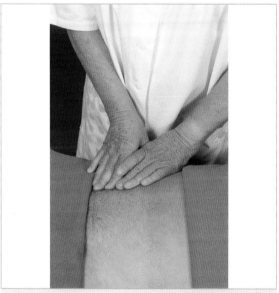

Fig. 10.74 (see Chapter 10.9.6) Treatment of the deep lymph vessels, right side.

11 Special Techniques

To treat various diseases, or skin or tissue changes, we use special techniques.

These are not different from the techniques described in the practical part of this textbook, but they have the typical characteristics of all techniques used in lymph drainage: circular skin movements, variable use of pressure during a circular movement, pressure adjusted to the clinical features of the individual, and pressure in the direction of lymph flow.

These techniques are combined with different movement and breathing exercises and with bandages, as necessary. The length of treatment depends on the symptoms.

Because of the way it works, there are many indications for manual lymph drainage. The training in the advanced classes enables the students to treat every pathology for which manual lymph drainage is indicated. Basically, any part of the body can be treated appropriately with the special techniques, as long as the characteristic general technique of manual lymph drainage is employed.

In general, special techniques are repeated many times because they are used very specifically for particular symptoms in the treatment of pathologies. For practice purposes, the special techniques, like the basic techniques, should be repeated at least three times.

When actually treating patients with certain pathologies, three repetitions are not enough; in the treatment context, the special techniques should be applied in a carefully targeted way and for longer.

> **Practice**
>
> *Repeat three times when practicing. Repeat more often when actually treating patients with specific pathologies.*

11.1 Special Techniques for the Head

11.1.1 Nose

2 and 2 fingers (index and middle finger) are placed at the side of the tip of the nose, one of them (the middle finger) on the nostrils. The order of the sequence is the same as in the basic technique. From the tip of the nose, 3 positions laterally; the same for the middle and root of the nose. After that, drain from the root of the nose to the nostrils. At least 3 positions, 5 circles per position (not shown).

Personal Notes

11.1.2 Eyes

Tear sacs: With two fingers, 3 positions, 5 circles per position.

Lower eyelid: If possible, the patient should look upward, as this allows better treatment of the lower lids. If this is too uncomfortable for the patient, or not possible for some other reason, the lower lids are treated with the eyes closed. With one finger, several positions, 5 circles per position.

Upper eyelid: The index finger of the therapist can rest on the eyebrow (support), while the upper lid is treated with the eyes closed, several positions, 5 circles per position.

Cranial to the eyeball: In the first position, the index finger is placed transversely between the upper lid and the eyebrow. The direction of push pressure is posterior and lateral. In the second and third position, the fingertips point toward the feet again. The push-pressure direction during this vertical finger position (this may be done using two fingers) is caudal and outward.

Personal Notes

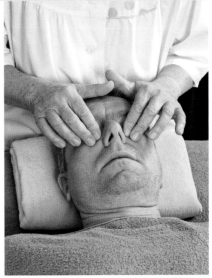
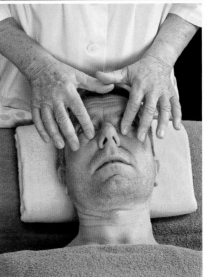
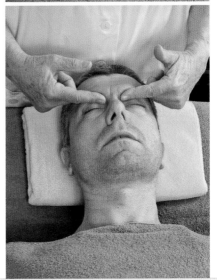

Fig. 11.1 (see Chapter 11.1.2)

11.1.3 Skull

Flat stationary circles in the area of the frontal hairline, at least 3 positions, 5 circles per position (not shown).

11.1.4 Ears

External ear: Index and middle finger are placed behind the ear as support and the thumb is in front of the ear. Thumb circles are performed in 2–3 imaginary lines, 5 circles per position. Work from the outside to the inside of the ear.

Personal Notes

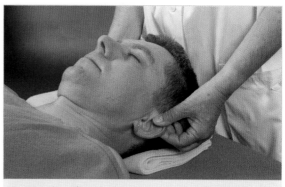

Fig. 11.2 (see Chapter 11.1.4) External ear: external line; position 1.

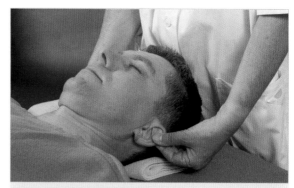

Fig. 11.3 (see Chapter 11.1.4) Position 2.

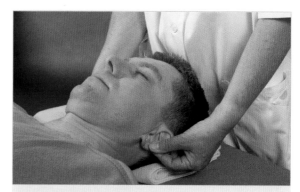

Fig. 11.4 (see Chapter 11.1.4) Position 3.

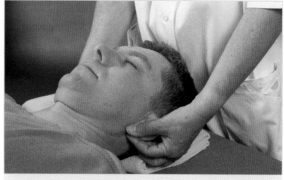

Fig. 11.5 (see Chapter 11.1.4) Position 4.

Auditory canal: Pressure into the auditory canal using the index, middle, or little finger.

Tragus: Thumb circles on the tragus with the index finger as support (not shown).

Around the ear: Stationary circles with flat extended fingers around the ear, several positions, 5 circles per position.

11.1.5 Intraoral Drainage (Not Shown)

The therapist stands on the right side of the patient.

Hard palate: The index or middle finger is placed on the hard palate. Work in a zigzag pattern back toward the soft palate, pressing up into the head, 5 times in each position, supporting the top of the head with the other hand.

Soft palate: The same as the treatment of the hard palate but with less pressure. Distracting motion on the root of the nose.

Cheeks: The extended index or middle finger is placed against the cheek from the inside. At the same time, the fingers of the other hand are placed against the outside of the cheek and pressure is applied with the internal finger against light resistance from the external fingers.

Personal Notes

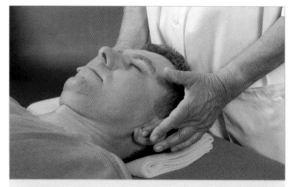

Fig. 11.6 (see Chapter 11.1.4) Auditory canal: pressure into the auditory canal using the middle finger.

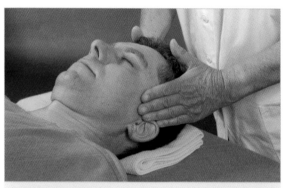

Fig. 11.7 (see Chapter 11.1.4) Around the ear: anterior.

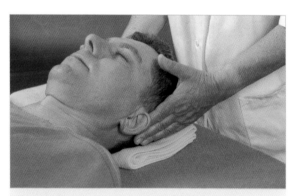

Fig. 11.8 (see Chapter 11.1.4) Around the ear: superior.

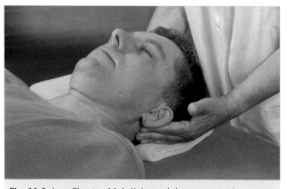

Fig. 11.9 (see Chapter 11.1.4) Around the ear: posterior.

11.2 Special Techniques for the Arm

11.2.1 Elbow

Thumb behind thumb, thumb circles on the forearm toward the epicondyle (not shown).

With **8 fingers** ("soldiers") on the tendons of the extensors and flexors, transverse friction (not shown).

Stationary circles with **flat fingers** placed around the lateral or medial epicondyle (not shown).

Pump technique on the elbow with movement of the elbow.

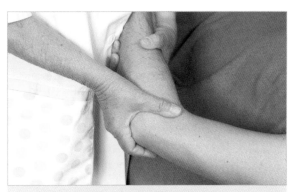

Fig. 11.10 (see Chapter 11.2.1) Pump technique on the elbow while extending the arm.

11.2.2 Wrist (Not Shown)

With the finger pads, pressing into the wrist with and without movement of the joint.

Pump technique on the joint, moving the joint.

Intensive thumb circles over the joint.

"Soldiers" technique: work with the finger pads between ulna and radius.

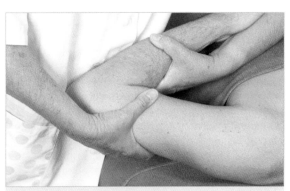

Fig. 11.11 (see Chapter 11.2.1) Pump technique on the elbow while flexing the arm.

Personal Notes

11.3 Special Techniques for the Leg

11.3.1 Knee

Moving the patella: Medially, laterally, inferiorly, superiorly, and in a circle (not shown).

Palpating technique: ("Soldiers") along the border of the patella. Medially with the finger pads, laterally with the thumbs, push the border from above and below toward the opposite side (not shown).

Joint pump: Place the palm of the hand on the patella; apply circling pressure with the hand on the patella, pressure toward the table. The other hand supports the knee joint from below (not shown).

Joint space of the knee: Flex the knee and place the foot on the table; look for the joint space of the knee, press and release into the space with the finger pads, 3 positions, 5 × per position (not shown).

Pump technique on the knee with movement. Allow the bent leg to rotate externally. The therapist holds the calf with the hand closer to the patient and moves the knee into flexion and extension. The other hand pumps over the knee from distal to proximal.

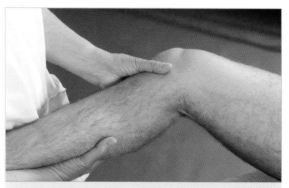

Fig. 11.12 (see Chapter 11.3.1) Pump technique over the knee with movement.

Personal Notes

11.3.2 Foot

"Soldiers" technique: Work with the fingers pads into the upper ankle joint while placing the thumbs on the sole of the foot to move the joint into dorsal extension, 5 × per position.

Pump over the sole and the dorsum of the foot simultaneously (not shown).

Pump over the ankle, in neutral position and with flexion and extension (5 pumps each) (not shown).

Pump medially or laterally over the malleoli using both hands at the same time. Position the patient accordingly (not shown).

Intensive thumb circles over the ankle joint (not shown).

Personal Notes

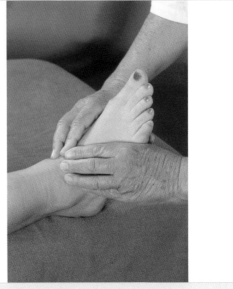

Fig. 11.13 (see Chapter 11.3.2) Working with the finger pads into the upper ankle joint.

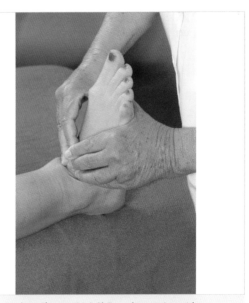

Fig. 11.14 (see Chapter 11.3.2) Dorsal extension with simultaneous pressure into the joint space.

11.4 Special Techniques for the Shoulder

The patient lies on the healthy side with the affected arm resting on the chest wall.

11.4.1 Mobilizing the Shoulder Blade Posteriorly

Practice

The therapist stands next to the table facing the patient. The therapist's arm that is closer to the patient's feet is pushed under the arm of the patient until they are elbow crease to elbow crease and the therapist's finger pads are on the medial border of the patient's scapula.

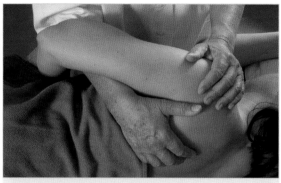

Fig. 11.15 (see Chapter 11.4.1) Finger pads are pushed underneath the medial border of the scapula.

Using the hand closer to the patient's head, the therapist grasps the shoulder joint and moves the shoulder in a circular motion dorsomedially and caudally. At the same time, the finger pads of the other hand are pushed underneath the medial border of the scapula. The finger pads travel up and down the medial border of the scapula.

Personal Notes

11.4.2 Mobilizing the Shoulder Blade Anteriorly

(Not shown).

The thumb of the therapist's hand that is closer to the feet is placed on the border of the latissimus dorsi and the teres major, caudal to the axilla. Using the contact on the cranial border of the scapula, the hand closer to the patient's head moves the scapula in a circular motion inferiorly and anteriorly. The thumb placed in the area of the latissimus dorsi and teres major does not move but provides resistance, so that the lateral scapula border and the latissimus dorsi move over the thumb. During this manipulation, the flexed arm of the patient is moved as well, reaching as much as 90-degree flexion.

Personal Notes

11.4.3 Glenohumeral Mobilization

Same starting position (SP) as before. Now the patient's arm is moved beyond 90 degrees into maximum flexion–elevation. The thumb remains the counterbalance, which creates a sort of resisted mobilization of the glenohumeral joint.

11.4.4 Searching for Painful Points: Patient in the Lateral Position (Not Shown)

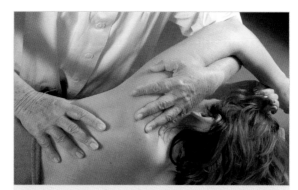

Fig. 11.16 (see Chapter 11.4.3) Glenohumeral mobilization.

Practice

Same SP as the technique above, patient's arm is relaxed on therapist's arm.

Additional Information

If the painful points are located, they are treated with flat fingers, using stationary circles with pressure and zero phase without inflicting any pain. The goal of the treatment of painful points is to act analgesically and to relax. It is important to take into account the direction of lymph flow when applying the stationary circles.

Descending part of the trapezius and supraspinatus: With both hands, fingers at a steep angle to the skin ("soldiers" technique), simultaneously palpate from the neck to the shoulder joint.

Supraspinatus: Palpate with the middle finger in the angle between scapular spine and clavicle, in the corner of the supraspinous fossa (furthest lateral). If pain is present, treat with pressure and zero phase, exerting pressure through the middle finger.

Deltoid: Palpate the border and the belly of the muscle with both hands simultaneously, fingers at a steep angle to the skin ("soldiers").

Biceps: Palpate the long biceps tendon between the major and minor tuberosity with the index or the middle finger. The other hand, placed dorsally, provides resistance.

Triceps and **teres major:** Palpate the area of the posterior axillary fold with the finger pads. The other hand, placed ventrally, provides resistance.

Personal Notes

11.4.5 Searching for Painful Points: Patient in Supine Position (Not Shown)

Additional Information

If the painful points or structures close to the joints are very sensitive, they are treated with a flat technique, pressure, and zero phase. The goal of the treatment of painful points is to act analgesically and to relax. It is important to take into account the direction of lymph flow when applying the stationary circles.

Sternoclavicular joint: Palpate the joint space and the structures around the joint. The joint space is located by placing the palpating index or middle finger on the area of the joint (near the jugular fossa), while moving the shoulder back and forth. The range of motion can be felt in the sternoclavicular joint space.

Acromioclavicular joint: Palpate the joint space and the structures around the joint with one or two fingers.

Head of the humerus: Palpate the structures in the area of the head of the humerus with the finger pads of both hands simultaneously.

Pectoralis major: Palpate the origin of the greater pectoral on the sternum and the clavicle with the finger pads of both hands simultaneously.

Pectoralis minor: Palpate the area of the coracoid process and the third to fifth ribs with the finger pads of both hands simultaneously.

Personal Notes

11.5 Special Techniques for the Back

11.5.1 Intercostal Spaces (Not Shown)

Practice

The patient is prone.

"Soldiers" technique in the intercostal spaces: Direction of pressure is inward (into the thorax). Simultaneous circles with both hands releasing toward the spine. The therapist stands facing the patient's feet. All intercostal spaces are treated; 5 × per position.

11.5.2 Extensors of the Spine (Not Shown)

Flat stationary circles with flat fingers over the extensors of the spine: Direction of pressure is down (into the table) similar to the "soldiers" technique on the spine. Circles toward the head. Several positions, 5 × per position (not shown).

Personal Notes

11.6 Special Techniques for the Hips

11.6.1 Standing behind the Patient

Practice

The patient lies on the healthy side with support for the head. A pillow is placed between the knees. The therapist stands behind the patient.

Gluteals: Alternating rotary technique from the iliac crest to the gluteal crease in 3 lines and back.

Deep abdominal lymph nodes: The patient turns slightly toward the therapist, taking a position between supine and lateral. The therapist places the fingers of both hands flat next to each other on the pubic bone, next to the most caudal part of the rectus abdominis. Without applying pressure, the skin is moved caudally, followed by pressure and pushed inward and cranially in the manner of a **stationary circle.** Direction of pressure is toward the cisterna chyli. 3 × (not shown).

Adductors and hamstring: Bend the leg and rotate it externally if possible without causing pain to the patient. The leg is stabilized in this position by tucking the foot under the knee or opposite lower leg, allowing relaxation. Palpate using **stationary circles** with both hands simultaneously, beginning distally on the ischiocrurals (hamstrings) and on the adductors. The hands move proximally until one hand reaches the ischial tuberosity (origin of the ischiocrurals) and the other the adductor longus (origin on the pubic bone).

First, palpate the origin of the adductor longus for possible tenderness. If it is tender, treat with flat technique, pressure, and zero phase. One hand stabilizes the leg by holding the knee. Then palpate the origin of the adductor magnus and posterior thigh muscles at the ischial tuberosity with the other hand. If tender, treat.

Personal Notes

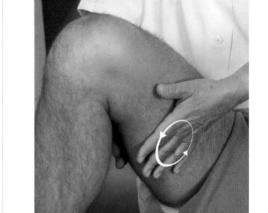

Fig. 11.17 (see Chapter 11.6.1) Alternating rotary technique over the gluteals.

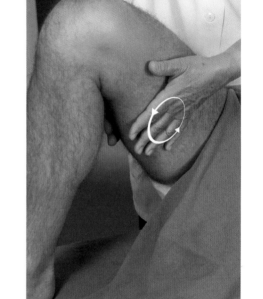

Fig. 11.18 (see Chapter 11.6.1) Stationary circles, adductors, and ischiocrurals (hamstrings): several positions.

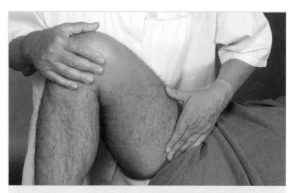

Fig. 11.19 (see Chapter 11.6.1) Palpation of the adductor origin; if it is tender, use flat stationary circles.

11.6.2 Standing in Front of the Patient

Practice

The therapist changes sides and now stands in front of the patient. The patient remains lying on the healthy side.

Gluteus medius: The therapist palpates the border of the muscle using the pads of the fingers of the hand closer to the head, while the hand closer to the feet flexes and extends the leg in the hip joint (not shown).

   Greater trochanter: The therapist palpates around the greater trochanter without moving the leg, using the "soldiers" technique (not shown).

Practice

If palpation reveals tender areas, they are treated with stationary circles or pump-push techniques.

11.6.3 Standing Next to the Patient

Practice

The patient is supine and the therapist changes sides again.

Iliac: Palpate the iliac in the area of the iliac crest with the finger pads of both hands. If the muscle is tender, it is treated with a sawing motion or with pressure and zero phase (not shown).

   Symphysis: Palpate the structures around the symphysis and the symphysis itself, the flexible juncture between the right and left pubic bones (not shown).

   Rectus abdominis: Palpate the insertion of the rectus abdominis on the pubic bone. In case of tenderness, treat with stationary circles (not shown).

   Pectineus: Palpate the insertion of the pectineus (which is an adductor), looking for tender areas.

Adductor canal: **Stationary circles** with the finger pads are used in the adductor canal from distal to proximal, applying light pressure ("soldiers technique" 3 positions, 3 circles per position.

   Adductors: Large areas of the adductors, located on the medial aspect of the thigh, are treated with the pump-push technique, both hands alternating, using increasing intensity.

Practice

If the palpated points are sensitive, they are treated with a flat technique, pressure, and zero phase. The goal of the treatment of painful points is to act analgesically and to relax. It is important to take into account the direction of lymph flow when applying the stationary circles.

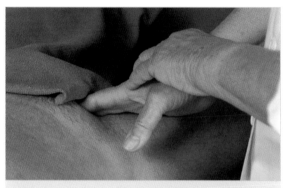

Fig. 11.20 (see Chapter 11.6.3) Palpation of the pectineus.

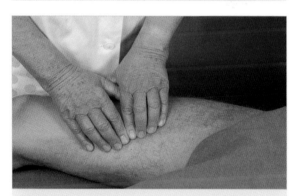

Fig. 11.21 (see section 11.6.3) Treatment of the adductor canal with the finger pads.

Personal Notes

11.7 Special Techniques for the Chest

11.7.1 Intercostal Spaces

Practice

The therapist stands next to the patient, looking toward the patient's head.

"Soldiers" technique in the intercostal spaces: Direction of pressure is inward (into the thorax), circles toward the sternum, several positions per intercostal space, from lateral to medial, 5 × per position (not shown).

11.7.2 Breathing Technique

Practice

The therapist stands next to the patient, looking toward the patient's feet.

Bronchitis technique: Eight finger pads are placed on the right or left costal arch. During expiration, the wrist moves the skin toward the fingers and the fingertips wrap around and underneath the costal arch. During this technique, the patient's legs are bent with the feet placed flat on the table. During inspiration, the fingers relax.

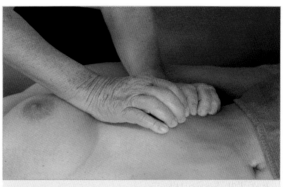
Fig. 11.22 (see Chapter 11.7.2) Bronchitis technique, inspiration phase.

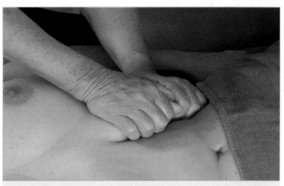
Fig. 11.23 (see Chapter 11.7.2) Bronchitis technique, expiration phase.

Personal Notes

11.8 Special Techniques for the Abdomen

The basic purpose of the techniques listed below is to stimulate the lymphangiomotoricity of the deep abdominal lymph vessels. The techniques have a strong inward effect on the abdomen, but they should not be painful. The patient's breathing rhythm has to be observed. If the therapist feels the pulsation of the abdominal aorta, downward pressure is not increased any further.

11.8.1 Wide Pelvis

"Nine" technique: The therapist places his/her hands one on top of the other on the patient's navel. The patient is asked to breathe deeply in and out once. During expiration, the therapist presses with the left hand over the metacarpophalangeal joints of the other hand, applying progressively deeper pressure, supinating at the end of each press. During inspiration, the therapist does not return entirely to zero, but keeps exerting light pressure to move deeper into the abdomen during the next expiration phase. Nine positions are treated on the abdomen, 5 × per position.

11.8.2 Narrow Pelvis

"Five" technique: For technique and performance, see "nine" technique (above). In a narrow pelvis, only 5 positions are treated, 5 × per position.

Personal Notes

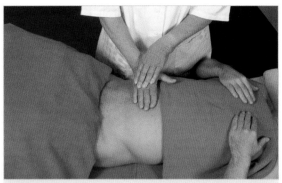

Fig. 11.24 (see Chapter 11.8) "Nine" technique, position on the navel.

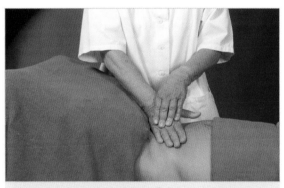

Fig 11.25 (see Chapter 11.8) "Nine" technique, position between the navel and the pubic bone.

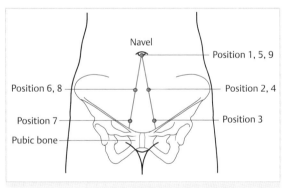

Fig. 11.26 The nine positions of the "nine" technique.

12 Treatment Model for Secondary Lymphedema

The following two models illustrate the textbook treatment of secondary lymphedema of the upper and lower extremities. It is assumed that important lymph node groups are not functioning. In this treatment, these lymph node groups are omitted or are bypassed using special techniques. These models cannot be applied in general to all cases of secondary lymphedema. The therapist must always search for the particular cause of the lymphedema in the individual case.

It is best to repeat each technique three times when practicing. In actual treatments, techniques should be targeted to the clinical features of the case, and should be repeated more often.

Additional Information

A treatment concept can only be put together once the cause of the lymphedema has been identified. Successful treatment of lymphedema is based on targeting the clinical features of the case.

12.1 Treatment of Secondary Lymphedema of the Arm

A patient who has undergone surgery for breast cancer with axillary lymphadenectomy on one side only, no complications, with or without radiation.

Practice

The patient is supine. The therapist stands on the patient's operated side.

12.1.1 Lymph Nodes of the Neck (Not Shown)

Stationary circles: profundus to terminus.
Stationary circles: occiput to terminus.

12.1.2 Healthy Breast (Not Shown)

Stationary circles in the area of the axillary lymph nodes.
  Pump-push across the mammary gland.
  Stationary circles in the intercostal spaces (spread fingers).
  "Soldiers" technique on the insertion of the ribs at the sternum.

Personal Notes

12.1.3 Affected Breast

Additional Information

Every technique performed on the affected side must move across the horizontal caudal or the vertical watershed following the anastomoses, so the lymph-obligatory load is always transported into a properly functioning drainage area.

Windshield wipers: Both hands are placed with flat fingers below the clavicle and above any scar. The skin is moved, both hands alternating, in continuous circles to the contralateral side.

Rotary technique: Above and below any scar, toward the healthy side (not shown).

Rotary technique: Across the horizontal caudal watershed into the inguinal drainage area; start at the watershed (not shown).

"Soldiers" technique: On the insertion of the ribs at the sternum (affected side) with light pressure toward the sternum and circles toward the head (not shown).

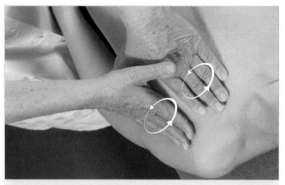

Fig. 12.1 (see Chapter 12.1.3) "Windshield wipers" away from the axilla.

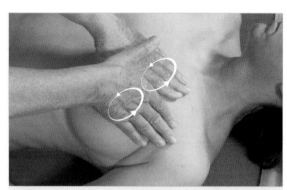

Fig. 12.2 (see Chapter12.1.3) "Windshield wipers" below the clavicle.

Personal Notes

12.1.4 Treatment of the Edematous Arm

Additional Information

The axillary drainage area is no longer functioning due to the removal or radiation of some or many axillary lymph nodes.

Thumb circles: The patient's arm is lifted and tucked under the therapist's lateral arm. From an imaginary line running from the middle of the axilla to the medial epicondyle, perform thumb circles with both hands simultaneously toward the dorsal aspect of the upper arm, beginning at the axilla.

Pump-push technique: The arm is placed back on the table. From the lateral aspect of the upper arm, over the deltoid, to the terminus on the same side (not shown).

Personal Notes

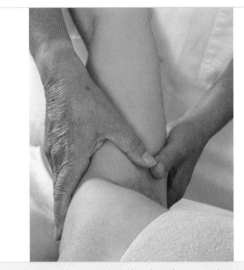

Fig. 12.3 (see Chapter12.1.4) Thumb circles proceeding laterally from the middle of the axilla, starting position.

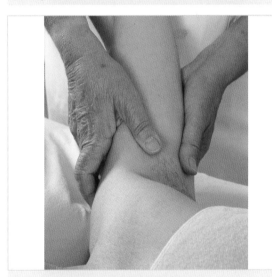

Fig. 12.4 (see Chapter12.1.4) "Push phase."

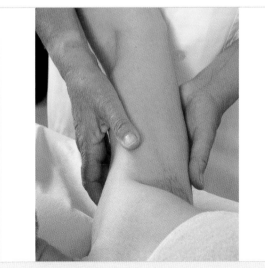

Fig. 12.5 (see Chapter12.1.4) "Zero phase."

Large-area pump technique over the elbow to the terminus (not shown).

Spiraling in the elbow crease from medial to lateral, with a lateral pull, with transitions to the pump technique toward the terminus (not shown).

Edema technique on the forearm: In the case of hard edema (fibrosis), begin proximally, 5 × per position. In the case of soft edema, begin distally and advance proximally.

Wrist: Hand and finger treatment as in the basic technique. Large-area techniques (pump technique over the hand) complement hand and finger treatment (not shown).

Drain the arm again from distal to proximal up to terminus (not shown).

> ### Practice
>
> *In edema treatment, large-area techniques are preferred over small-area techniques. Small-area techniques are technique variations.*

Personal Notes

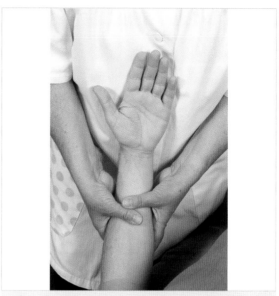

Fig. 12.6 (see Chapter12.1.4) Edema technique on the forearm, zero phase.

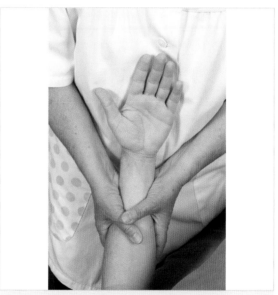

Fig. 12.7 (see Chapter12.1.4) Edema technique on the forearm, push phase.

12.1.5 Affected Breast (Not Shown)

Additional Information

Every technique performed on the affected side must move across the horizontal caudal or the vertical watershed, so that the lymph-obligatory load is always transported into a properly functioning drainage area.

Windshield wiper: Both hands are placed with flat fingers below the clavicles and above any scar. The skin is moved, hands alternating, in continuous circles to the contralateral side.

Rotary technique: Above and below any scar, in direction of a properly functioning drainage area, across the vertical watershed toward the healthy side (not shown).

Rotary technique: Starting at the horizontal caudal watershed moving into the inguinal drainage area (not shown).

"Soldiers" technique: On the insertion of the ribs at the sternum on the affected side, with light pressure toward the sternum and circles toward the head (not shown).

12.1.6 Back (Not Shown)

Practice

The patient turns onto her healthy side. The therapist changes sides.

Alternating rotary technique from the posterior axillary fold across the spine to the healthy side of the back.

Intercostal spaces are treated intensely with 8 fingers.

Flat fingers treat the extensors of the spine. Pressure is inward (toward the body), circles toward the head.

Practice

Place the affected arm along the side of the body.

Pump and push toward the shoulder, beginning at the hand, turning into rotary technique along the border of the trapezius crossing the vertical watershed (with the whole hand).

Bandage with proper padding.

Personal Notes

12.2 Treatment of Secondary Lymphedema of the Leg

A patient with abdominal cancer who has undergone lymphadenectomy in the lesser pelvis or the groin, with or without radiation therapy.

> **Practice**
>
> *The patient is supine.*

12.2.1 Lymph Nodes of the Neck (Not Shown)

Stationary circles from profundus to terminus.
  Stationary circles from occiput to terminus.

12.2.2 Axillary Lymph Nodes (Not Shown)

The therapist stands behind the patient's head.
  Stationary circles on the lateral thoracic wall in the area of the anterior axillary fold.
  Stationary circles in the axilla.
  Stationary circles on the medial aspect of the upper arm.

12.2.3 Abdominal Skin

Rotary technique over the skin of the abdomen. Work via lympho-lymphatic anastomoses using the rotary technique, from the inguinal to the axillary drainage area. Starting at the horizontal watershed, moving in several steps caudally.

Personal Notes

12.2.4 Treatment of the Edematous Leg from the Front

Windshield wiper and rotary technique. The thigh is treated with the windshield wiper technique (see treatment of the breast under "Treatment of Secondary Lymphedema of the Arm") from the medial aspect (adductors) to the lateral aspect (iliotibial tract). In the starting position (SP) on the medial aspect of the thigh, the therapist holds one hand in slight ulnar abduction and the other one in slight radial abduction. The hands move alternately, using push-pressure and zero phase, on an imaginary line from medial to lateral. On the lateral aspect of the thigh (iliotibial tract), the rotary technique is used toward the axillary drainage area, keeping one hand behind the other; the lateral hand starts.

Personal Notes

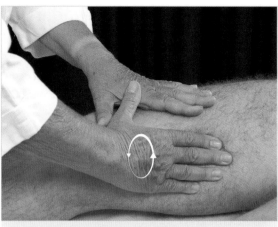

Fig. 12.8 (see Chapter 12.2.4) "Windshield wipers," push-pressure phase with the right hand.

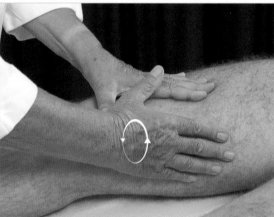

Fig. 12.9 (see Chapter 12.2.4) "Windshield wipers," starting position on the medial aspect of the thigh, zero phase.

The knee is treated using the basic technique. In addition, large-area techniques are applied, or "double pump" with two hands from medial to lateral (not shown).

Edema technique on the lower leg. The edema technique is applied, advancing if the edema is soft, applying the pump technique on the shin and the scoop technique on the calf.

Additional Information

If fibrosis is present, edema techniques are performed on one spot, without advancing, and with considerably more pressure. Treatment begins proximally.

Achilles tendon, ankle joint, dorsum of the foot, and lymph sea are treated using the basic technique. In addition, large-area techniques are applied (not shown).

Finally, the entire leg is drained proximally, from medial to lateral above the knee (windscreen wipers), and then drainage continues over the iliotibial tract to the axillary drainage area with rotary technique (not shown).

Practice

The patient is prone.

Personal Notes

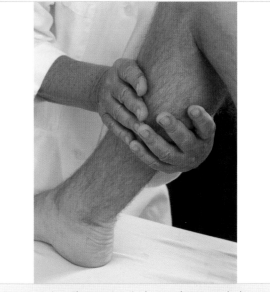

Fig. 12.10 (see Chapter 12.2.4) Edema technique on the lower leg, medial aspect.

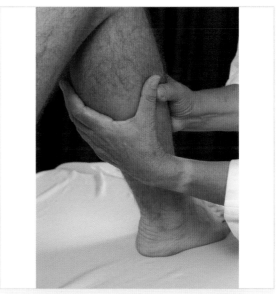

Fig. 12.11 (see Chapter 12.2.4) Edema technique on the lower leg, lateral aspect

12.2.5 Quadratus Lumborum (Not Shown)

Stationary circles in the area between the 12th rib and the iliac crest.

12.2.6 "Soldiers" Technique (Not Shown)

"Soldiers" paravertebrally on the sacrum and the lumbar spine.

12.2.7 Skin of the Buttocks (Not Shown)

Rotary technique: The skin of the buttocks is drained via lympho-lymphatic anastomoses into the axillary drainage area, starting at the horizontal watershed.

Personal Notes

12.2.8 Treatment of the Edematous Leg from Behind

Windshield wiper and rotary technique: The thigh is treated with the windshield wiper technique (see "Treatment of the Edematous Leg from the Front") from the medial aspect (adductors) to the lateral aspect (iliotibial tract). In the SP on the medial aspect of the thigh, the therapist holds one hand in slight ulnar abduction and the other one in slight radial abduction. The hands move alternately, using push-pressure and zero phase, on an imaginary line from medial to lateral. On the lateral aspect of the thigh (iliotibial tract), rotary technique is used toward the axillary drainage area.

The popliteal area is treated with flat pump technique and thumb circles (not shown).

The lower leg is treated with the soft edema technique from distal to proximal if soft edema is present.

Additional Information

If fibrotic changes are present in the lower leg, use fibrosis techniques in a stationary circular manner working from proximal to distal, 5 × each.

The Achilles tendon is treated with thumb circles and pump technique.

The sole of the foot is treated with pump technique and with thumb circles simultaneously and alternately.

Finally, the entire leg is drained proximally. On the distal third of the thigh, use windshield wipers moving laterally and then proximally along the iliotibial tract and crossing the caudal watershed into the axillary drainage area.

Bandage with proper padding.

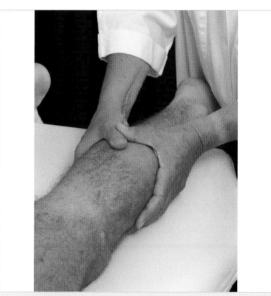

Fig. 12.12 (see Chapter 12.2.8) Soft edema technique from distal to proximal.

Personal Notes

Part IV

Complementary Treatments

IV

13 Complementary Treatments

13.1 Decongestion and Maintenance Phase

Conventional medicine recognizes combined decongestive therapy (CDT) as the treatment for lymphedema. CDT is divided into a decongestion phase (phase 1) and a maintenance phase (phase 2). Specific conditions during the two phases require specific complementary treatments. Not every patient with a prescription for manual lymph drainage is a candidate for CDT therapy. In some cases, a diagnosis requiring manual lymph drainage can be combined with certain complementary treatments, and sometimes manual lymph drainage alone is helpful.

The pillars of lymphedema treatment during the decongestion phase are as follows:
- Skin care.
- Manual lymph drainage.
- Bandages.
- Therapeutic exercises and respiratory therapy.

Procedures of the maintenance phase vary only slightly from the decongestion phase, but the order of importance of the individual therapies is different:
- Skin care.
- Compression stockings.
- Therapeutic exercises and respiratory therapy.
- Manual lymph drainage. Q 28

13.1.1 Phase 1: Inpatient Decongestion Phase

For decongestion treatment, patients are usually hospitalized in a lymphedema clinic that specializes in CDT. The duration of the stay varies from 3 to 6 weeks. During this time, the patient receives lymph drainage treatment once or twice a day for 1 hour. The duration of stay and frequency of treatment depend on the diagnosis and stage of the lymphedema. Therapy sessions end with bandaging of the edematous extremity. The patients have the opportunity to rest afterward and then take part in exercise groups, which may include edema exercises, Nordic walking, dance therapy, or bicycling. Before the next manual lymph drainage treatment, patients take part in water exercises, where they move without bandages or "only" wearing compression stockings.

> **Note**
>
> *For therapy to be successful, it is crucial that the edematous extremity is bandaged or the patient wears the proper compression stocking during movement therapy.*

During the inpatient phase, patients learn how to bandage themselves. If there is still time after the therapy sessions described earlier, patients can take up the offer of autogenic training, Feldenkrais groups, or similar activities, in order to learn to deal with personal stress. In our experience—although we have no scientific proof to support this—stress has a negative effect on lymphedema.

During the inpatient phase, the therapy center offers various evening classes for lymphedema patients relating to general rules of everyday behavior, nutrition, and the development of lymphedema. Evening group sessions with specialists trained in psychology, who also offer individual sessions, and evening classes on "cooking for a lymphedema patient" round off the program at the Wittlinger Therapy Center in Walchsee in the Austrian Tirol, a specialist lymphology clinic.

History taking by physicians trained in lymphology, daily rounds by physicians, medication monitoring, interdisciplinary therapy team conferences (both regular and as required by special patient problems), medical attendance in case of emergencies, the use of objective measurement methods (Perometer), and treatment of comorbidities are all part of standard everyday practice at our lymphology center. When lymphedema patients are discharged, they are supplied with custom-fitted arm or leg compression stockings and receive a medical report for their treating physician.

13.1.2 Phase 1: Outpatient Decongestion Phase

In certain cases, it is possible to treat the patient during the decongestion phase as an outpatient. Usually, this is done in a practice specializing in the treatment of lymphedema.

Outpatient decongestion entails a variety of difficulties with regard to edema patient care. Without wishing to question the abilities of our physiotherapy colleagues, the comprehensive care possible in inpatient decongestion therapy cannot be given in the outpatient setting. Daily manual lymph drainage and proper bandaging are the top priorities if edema treatment is to be successful.

The biggest problems in treating lymphedema patients in the outpatient setting, in both the decongestion and the maintenance phase, are the following:

- Receiving a proper prescription. Instructions may be missing as to:
  - The duration and frequency of the manual lymph drainage treatment.
  - Bandaging.
  - The use of bandaging materials, including the necessary padding.
  - The duration and frequency of any additional group or individual therapy sessions.

- Lack of proper bandaging materials, including the necessary padding, in outpatient physiotherapy or massage practices.
- Inadequate physical therapeutic examination.
- Difficulties in monitoring patient compliance.
- Too little time or none for group therapy sessions, seminars, etc.
- Lack of psychological care.
- Lack of information and instruction about nutrition and food preparation.

13.1.3 Phase 2: Maintenance Phase

Patients being discharged from a lymphology clinic and/or from outpatient lymphology rehabilitation are usually supplied with custom-made, flat-knitted compression stockings. Recommendations for further treatment, or the treatment report of the therapist, are sent to the referring physician.

Physical therapists or massage therapists who have successfully completed the appropriate 4-week manual lymph drainage training are qualified to treat lymphedema patients appropriately.

Therapy sessions take place once or twice a week. During these sessions, the therapist must ensure that the patient wears the compression stocking and carries out the exercises given as homework.

When wearing the compression stocking, it is important that it should fit properly. The patient should also be shown exercises that support lymphatic return. These exercises should not be too complicated. To achieve the support of lymphatic return needed in the leg edema patient, it is often enough just to walk with the compression stocking on. Patients with arm edema can activate the arm muscles by going walking or hiking with Nordic walking or simple walking sticks. Every arm movement with the stick promotes lymphatic return from the edematous upper extremity—with the compression stocking on. The main goal in phase 2, the maintenance phase, is to uphold the achievements of phase 1, the decongestion phase. Treatments with manual lymph drainage support

the maintenance of the therapeutic success of the decongestion phase. Q 34

13.2 Skin Care

In an adult, the skin covers an area of approximately 2 m². A distinction is made between epidermis, dermis, and the subcutaneous fatty tissue. The acid mantle of the skin is produced in the epidermis.

Lymphedema stretches the skin, which among other problems causes a disturbance in the acid mantle. Lymph cysts—enlargements of initial lymph vessels in the skin that are filled with lymph—may form. These cysts can burst or become damaged, leading to the formation of a lymph fistula with flow of lymph to the outside. This may result in viral or fungal infections. The tissue pressure is increased and so the nutritional supply of the epidermis becomes inadequate. Protein congestion in the skin leads to the activation of fibroblasts and hence to fibrosis. Pachyderma and hyperkeratosis may result as well.

Edema, or compression with short-stretch bandages or compression stockings, causes particular stress on the skin, which requires treatment. The material of the bandages and the stockings absorbs moisture and oil, meaning that the protective layer of the skin is at increased risk of infection. Regular use of a pH-neutral cream that does not contain alcohol or perfume is an important precaution. We recommend nourishing the skin approximately 1 hour before each treatment or in the evening. There are always some patients who regard this additional effort as a nuisance. However, this "work" can also be looked at as something positive. The patient pays attention to his or her body and will notice any injuries, redness, or other irregularities that require immediate care.

In the Wittlinger Therapy Center, we use our in-house brand Celuvase, which improves blood flow, especially in the regional blood capillaries of the affected skin area.

13.3 Compression Therapy

13.3.1 Bandaging

When treating lymphedema, manual lymph drainage should always be followed by compression therapy with bandaging. This inhibits refilling of the edematous area. Once the edema has been successfully treated with manual lymph drainage, the skin is saggy and too "big"; the elastic properties of the connective tissue are no longer effective. The compression pressure of the bandage replaces the absent tissue pressure. The bandage pressure also alters the volume of the blood vessels, especially in the low-pressure venous system. There, the flow rate increases and any insufficiencies of the venous valves are compensated.

Bandages also act as a kind of external resistance against internal—subfascial—muscle contractions. In this way, every muscle contraction generates a "massaging" of the blood and lymph vessels in the rhythm of the contraction. This effect is called the muscle pump, and it has considerable impact on the venous and lymphatic return.

> ### Note
>
> *No edema treatment without bandaging afterward!*

In the Wittlinger Therapy Center/Dr. Vodder Academy, we use short- and long-stretch bandages for decongestion. For outpatient treatments, we also use bandaging techniques with short- and long-stretch material. In general, in inpatient treatment mostly short-stretch bandages are used. For certain lymphedema conditions, long- and short-stretch bandages are used simultaneously, depending on the clinical findings. For the success of the compression therapy, it is crucial that the bandage material is carefully adjusted to the individual patient and to the extremity being bandaged.

The bandage pressure on the extremities must stay within certain limits. Venous blood and lymph transport must be promoted, but the arterial blood flow must not become restricted.

Wear Time

In general, compression bandages are worn day and night. On days without manual lymph drainage treatment, the patient must apply the bandages himself or herself after daily personal care. In some exceptional cases, it is possible to elevate the extremity during the night and forego the compression.

Bandages should only be worn as long as they do not cause pain or discomfort that can be attributed to the bandaging itself.

Wear Time during Phase 1: Decongestion Phase of Combined Decongestive Therapy

During inpatient treatment in a clinic, bandages are worn the entire time between treatments. Clinic staffs are trained to ensure the wearing of bandages.

In outpatient decongestion, the manual lymph drainage/CDT therapist must consider the occupational requirements, family situation, and other circumstances of the lymphedema patient with regard to the application of bandages. For example, bandages on the foot cannot be too voluminous for the patient to wear shoes. Arm bandages must not limit mobility to the extent that the patient is impeded at work.

Wear Time during Phase 2: Maintenance Phase of Combined Decongestive Therapy

Once treatments take place at longer intervals, patients must be able to apply the bandages every day themselves. Optimally, they should put aside 2 hours in the evening, to include time for proper skin care. Therapists working in an outpatient practice must make sure that the patient understands and is able to perform the bandaging technique.

Technique

The bandage must always be adapted to the shape of the extremity. Particular anatomical features such as ankle, wrist, or loose subcutaneous connective tissue must be padded to achieve sufficient and, above all, even compression. Padding also increases the pressure on the tissue. The bandages are wound on in upward circles. The pressure characteristics of bandaging obey the La Place law. The pressure should decrease from distal to proximal, allowing lymph drainage flow away from the extremities.

Bandaging Material

Through the use of various bandaging materials, varying individual requirements can be met (▶ **Fig. 13.1**). For example, elastic bandaging materials (long-stretch bandages) increase the resting pressure, whereas more rigid materials (short-stretch bandages) increase the working pressure during muscular exertion of the edematous extremity. This is often a desired therapeutic effect in the treatment of lymphedema.

A distinction is made between long-stretch bandage materials (rubber elasticity) and short-stretch bandage materials (fabric elasticity).

Long-stretch materials develop high resting pressure because of their high recoil force and low working

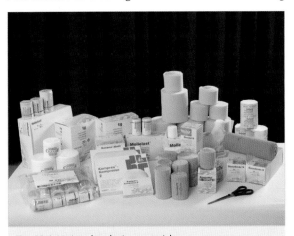

Fig. 13.1 Various bandaging materials.

pressure due to the low resistance produced by the rubber elasticity of the bandaging material against muscle contraction.

Short-stretch materials, on the other hand, develop low resting pressure because of their low recoil force and high working pressure due to the high resistance produced by the fabric elasticity of the bandaging material against muscle contraction.

The recoil force of the bandaging material has considerable influence on the resting and working pressure. Resting pressure and working pressure are two important terms with regard to the proper fitting of a bandage:

Resting pressure is the pressure that develops within the bandage when the patient does not move the edematous extremity, that is, does not contract muscles.

Working pressure is the pressure that develops within the bandage when the patient moves the edematous extremity, that is, contracts muscles.

▸ **Recoil force** is the force of the bandage by which it returns to the original state after being stretched. The higher the rubber content of the bandage, the stronger its effort to return from the stretched to the original state.
▸ **Long-stretch materials** have a high resting pressure and a low working pressure.
▸ **Short-stretch materials** have a low resting pressure and a hig h working pressure.

Bandage Pressure

In applying a bandage, the compression pressure must decrease from distal to proximal. The individual pressure sensitivity of the patient has to be taken into account.

To apply a bandage correctly, it is important to have an understanding of the La Place law. This law states that if the applied force remains the same while the radius of the extremity increases, the pressure decreases. In practice, this means that the compression pressure of a bandage or compression stocking is greatest when the radius is small. In many stage 1, and some light stage 2 lymphedemas, the extremity is narrower distally than proximally. In these cases, bandages are applied with the same distal and proximal pressure. Because of the La Place law, a pressure gradient is thus created from distal to proximal, which allows the lymph to drain from the edematous extremity.

The tightest that compression bandages may be applied is when blue discoloration of fingers and toes disappears with movement; if it does not, the bandages have been applied too tightly.

If the tips of fingers and toes turn white after the application of bandages, it must be assumed that the bandage pressure is too high and the arterial vessel system is being compressed. The bandage must be removed immediately and reapplied with less pressure.

Another significant reason for removing the bandage is if the patient complains about pain. The therapist has to be careful to differentiate when judging the patient's description of the pain, because at the start of compression therapy all patients experience the bandaging as uncomfortable and in some way painful. Discomfort is not a criterion for bandage removal. The therapist must proceed sensitively and ask the right questions to be able to distinguish between real pain, discomfort, and lack of compliance on the part of the patient.

Sequelae of bandages that are applied too tightly are as follows:
- Bursitis.
- Periostitis.
- Muscular pain and spasms.
- Skin abrasions.

Relative and/or Absolute Contraindications for Bandaging

Extremities are not bandaged in the case of the following:
1. *Erysipelas*: St. Anthony's fire, or cellulitis as erysipelas is also called, is a streptococcal infection of the skin. It is a frequent concomitant feature of lymphedema because the pathogens can enter through the smallest skin lesions. Patients must consult a physician as soon as possible and are treated with antibiotics. Manual lymph drainage treatment is only continued if acute symptoms have subsided during the use of antibiotics and inflammatory lesions have healed.
2. *Nerve damage and pain*: In patients with signs of paralysis or paresthesia, bandages must be applied with great caution. The examination should clarify the reason for nerve damage and pain. Bandages are applied in such a way that symptoms are not exacerbated.
3. *Diabetes*: Patients with diabetes mellitus frequently suffer from neurological disorders. The nerve damage depends on how long the patient has been diabetic and on his or her metabolic state. Symptoms of sensorimotor dysfunction caused by diabetic neuropathy include reduced tactile sensation, reduced sensation of pain and temperature, paresthesia (tingling), pain and burning sensations, reduced reflexes, and complete paralysis. It is obvious that bandaging must be done cautiously if some of these sensorimotor changes are present.
4. *Impaired arterial circulation*: Through certain pathophysiological mechanisms, occlusive arterial disease leads to malnutrition of the affected area. Obviously, given the known biomechanics, compressing an extremity in this way with bandages is contraindicated, since bandaging will compress the arterial lumina as well as those of the low-pressure (venous) system.
5. *Rheumatoid arthritis*: Patients with joint problems of this kind experience considerable pain in addition

to swelling of the joints and are therefore unable to tolerate bandages or compression stockings. However, manual lymph drainage is still indicated for this disorder (analgesic effect).

6. *Cardiac decompensation*: Patients with cardiac decompensation may have swollen legs. In cases of considerable decompensation, manual lymph drainage treatment for this type of edema is contraindicated because the resulting increase in lymph time volume, due to the stimulation of lymphangiomotoricity, overloads the already impaired heart through the elevated return of lymph-obligatory load. Lymphatic return also increases when extremities of patients with this disorder are bandaged. Bandaging alone can induce life-threatening conditions.

▶ Bandaging:
• Effect:
  – Substitutes for absence of tissue pressure.
  – Fibroses are loosened.
  – Increases lymphatic return.
  – Increases venous return.
• Materials:
  – Tubular bandage.
  – Short-stretch bandages with complete padding of the extremity.
  – Long-stretch bandages with partial padding of the extremity (padding consists of foam, cotton bandages, comprex, or similar material; the padding should not cause skin irritation or lesions).
  – Cotton bandages.
  – Special material such as adhesive bandages, etc.
• Area of application:
  – Upper extremities.
  – Lower extremities.
  – Abdominal and lumbar area.
  – Genital area.
• Time of application:
  – After every edema treatment without exception.
• Wear time:
  – In general, only as long as the patient does not experience pain or discomfort caused by the bandage.
  – During inpatient care, ideally until the next treatment.
  – During outpatient care if treatments are daily, also until the next treatment.
  – During outpatient care if treatments are less frequent, if possible (with self-bandaging by the patient) until the next treatment.
• Relative or absolute contraindications:
  – Erysipelas (cellulitis).
  – Nerve damage/pain.
  – Diabetes.
  – Impaired arterial circulation.
  – Open wounds (radiation ulcers).

Application of Bandages

Arms

• Begin with skin care (▶ **Fig. 13.2a,b**). In inpatient care, bandages are removed approximately 1 hour before treatment. The patient takes a shower, goes to the therapy session, and after the manual lymph drainage session the therapist performs the skin care.
• Dress the extremity with a cotton stocking (▶ **Fig. 13.3**).
• If necessary, apply finger bandages using 6-cm Mollelast bandages, reinforcing them with 4-cm Mollelast bandages (webbing; ▶ **Fig. 13.4a,b**).
• Pad the hand with foam (▶ **Fig. 13.5a–c**).

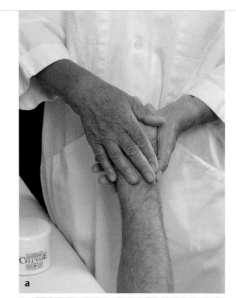
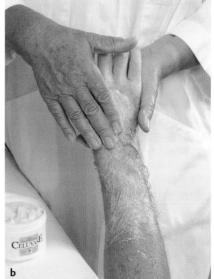

Fig. 13.2 (a,b) Follow-up skin care after manual lymph drainage treatment.

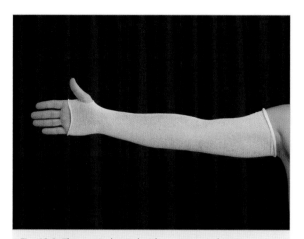

Fig. 13.3 The arm is dressed with a cotton stocking.

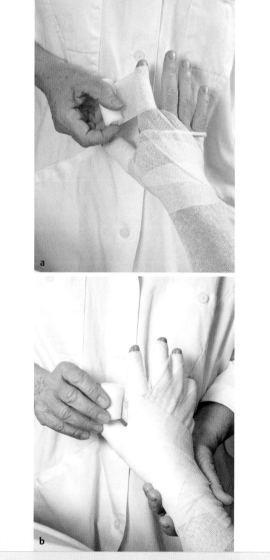

Fig. 13.4 Finger bandage **(a)** using 6-cm Mollelast and **(b)** reinforced with 4-cm Mollelast.

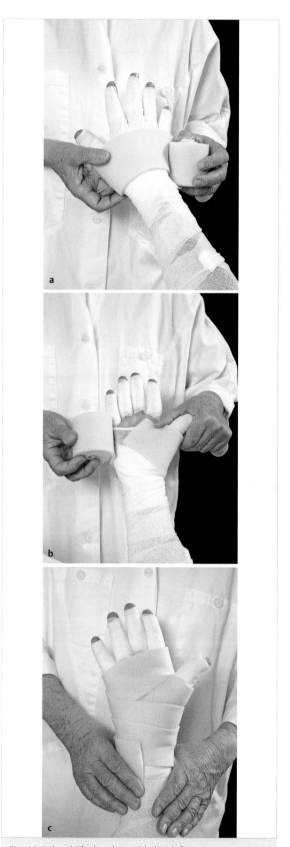

Fig. 13.5 **(a–c)** The hand is padded with foam.

115

When Using Short-stretch Material

- Pad the entire arm with foam of various thicknesses or other materials (▸ **Fig. 13.6**).
- Now apply a 6-cm short-stretch bandage to the hand (▸ **Fig. 13.7**).

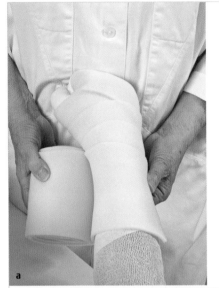

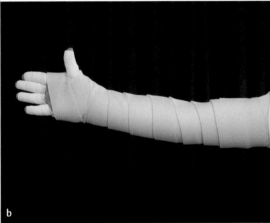

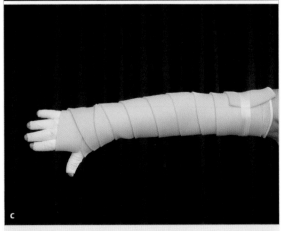

Fig. 13.6 (a–c) Padding of the entire arm.

- Follow with an 8-cm short-stretch bandage to the arm (▸ **Fig. 13.8**).
- Add a 10-cm short-stretch bandage to the arm (▸ **Fig. 13.9a,b**).
- Depending on the indication and how the patient feels, you may add further layers of 10-cm short-stretch bandages to reinforce the compression. Always start at the wrist.

When Using Long-stretch Material

- Dress the extremity with a cotton stocking.
- If necessary, apply finger bandaging.

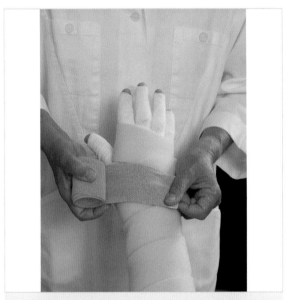

Fig. 13.7 Bandage using 6 cm-wide short-stretch bandage.

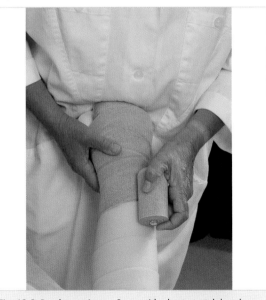

Fig. 13.8 Bandage using an 8-cm-wide short-stretch bandage.

- Pad the hand with foam.
- Apply a 6-cm long-stretch bandage to the hand (▶**Fig. 13.10**).

- Now apply an 8-cm long-stretch bandage to the arm (▶**Fig. 13.11**).
- Partially pad the elbow crease.
- Apply a 10-cm long-stretch bandage to the arm (▶**Fig. 13.12a,b**).

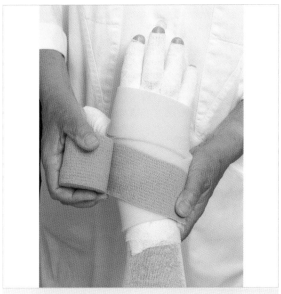

Fig. 13.10 Bandage using 6-cm long-stretch bandages.

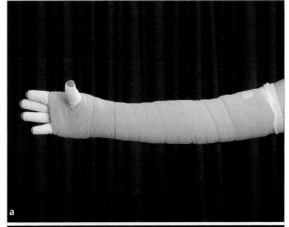

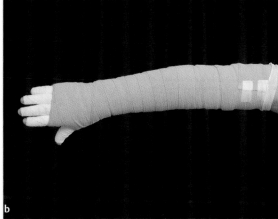

Fig. 13.9 (a,b) Bandage using 10-cm-wide short-stretch bandages.

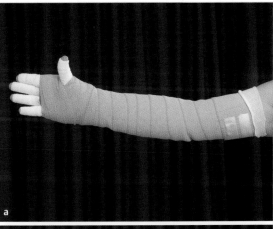

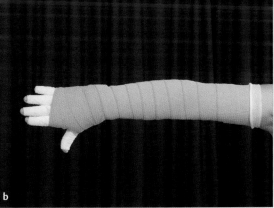

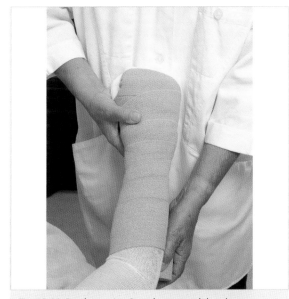

Fig. 13.11 Bandage using 8-cm long-stretch bandages.

Fig. 13.12 (a,b) Bandage using a 10-cm long-stretch bandage.

- If desired, you can add a 10-cm long-stretch bandage to reinforce the compression. Always start at the wrist.

Legs

- Begin with skin care (▶**Fig. 13.13**). In inpatient care, bandages are removed approximately 1 hour before treatment. The patient takes a shower, goes to the

therapy session, and after the manual lymph drainage session the therapist performs the skin care.
- Dress the extremity with a cotton stocking (▶**Fig. 13.14**).
- If necessary, follow with bandaging of the toes using 4-cm Mollelast bandages (▶**Fig. 13.15a,b**).
- When padding the foot, include the lymph sea and the malleoli (with kidneys) (▶**Fig. 13.16**).
- Pad the entire leg with foam or other materials (▶**Fig. 13.17a,b**).

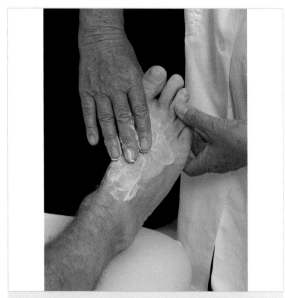

Fig. 13.13 Follow-up skin care after manual lymph drainage treatment.

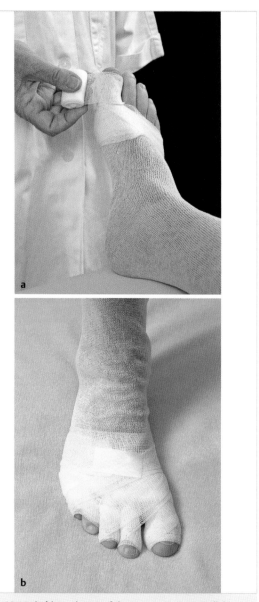

Fig. 13.15 (a,b) Bandaging of the toes using 4-cm Mollelast.

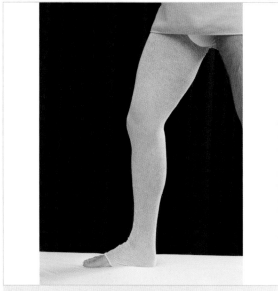

Fig. 13.14 The leg is dressed with a cotton stocking.

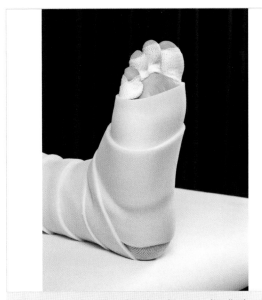

Fig. 13.16 Padding of the foot, lymph, sea, and malleoli.

- Depending on the size of the foot, apply an 8- or 10-cm short-stretch bandage to the foot. Begin in the area of the forefoot (▶Fig. 13.18a–c).
- Bandage the leg using 10-cm short-stretch bandages from the malleoli proximally (▶Fig. 13.19a–c).
- Ideal bandaging pressure is created when using at least five or six 10-cm short-stretch bandages of 10-m length each. The exact number of bandages used depends on the volume of the leg.
- Depending on the indication, the torso can be bandaged using one or more 20-cm long-stretch bandages without padding. Likewise the genitals using a 4-cm Mollelast bandage and two 6-cm Mollelast bandages (▶Fig. 13.20a,b).

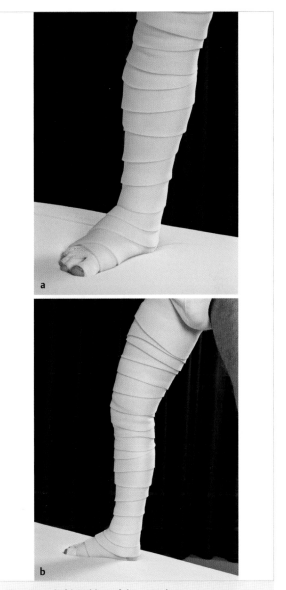

Fig. 13.17 (a,b) Padding of the entire leg.

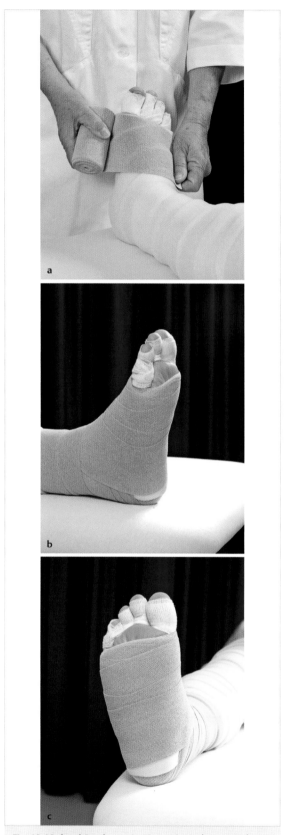

Fig. 13.18 (a–c) Bandage using 8- or 10-cm short-stretch bandages.

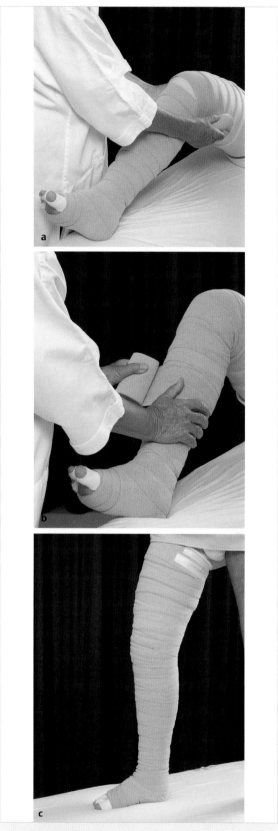

Fig. 13.19 (a–c) Bandage using a 10-cm short-stretch bandage from the malleoli proximally.

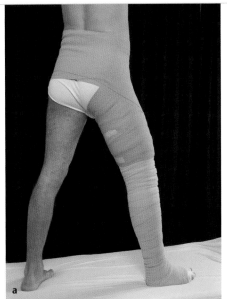

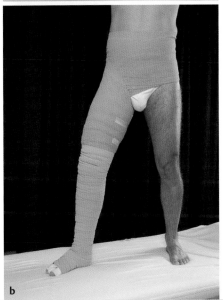

Fig. 13.20 (a,b) Bandaging of the torso using a 20-cm long-stretch bandage without padding.

Questions and Answers

Whether they work in inpatient or—especially—outpatient care, therapists often encounter questions from patients about bandaging. Compression therapy requires great discipline from patients. If the goal of inpatient or outpatient lymphedema therapy is to be reached, it is essential that they collaborate well. Motivating the patient to constantly be "wrapping up" the edematous leg or arm requires much sensitivity and persuasiveness on the part of the therapist. Here are some important

questions and possible answers that will help prepare you for practice:

- "Do I have to wear the bandages at night?"
  - "It is best if you can. If you have pain or cannot sleep with the bandages, you should remove them, but you must put them on again immediately when you get up in the morning."
- "How do I clean the bandages?"
  - "Manufacturers offer special detergents. You can also use a regular mild detergent. If possible, wash bandages by hand. Do not put them in the dryer."
- "What do I wear while I am cleaning the bandages?"
  - "It is best to have two sets of bandages. If that is not possible, wear your compression stocking."
- "Are bandages better than a custom-fitted compression stocking?"
  - "Bandages are always better than a compression stocking because their fit can be accurately adjusted to the extremity."
- "Is it necessary to elevate the bandaged arm?"
  - "If you can sleep with the arm elevated, you should do so. During the day, elevate the arm whenever possible."
- "Will my muscles waste away if I am always wearing the bandage?"
  - "No, because we encourage you to exercise while wearing the bandages. These muscle contractions not only counteract muscle wasting but also encourage venous and lymphatic reflux."
- "Is it better to use short- or long-stretch bandages?"
  - "This depends on the edema and the individual symptoms. It differs from patient to patient."

13.3.2 Compression Stockings

In the maintenance phase, compression therapy is primarily provided by custom-fitted compression stockings. Bandaging the edematous extremity becomes secondary. However, bandages may be used even during the maintenance phase to reinforce the compression pressure of the stockings, for example, during athletic activities or long flights. Like compression bandages, compression stockings are usually worn throughout the day.

If the applied force remains constant and the radius of the extremity increases, the pressure decreases proximally (La Place law). The pressure of compression stockings runs from 100% distal to 40% proximal. For this reason, they must be custom fitted with reference to the length and circumference of the edema. There are four uniformly regulated compression classes to choose from, depending on the severity of the lymphedema (**Table 13.1**).

Recent research has shown that after only 3 months the compression pressure of compression class 2 stockings has changed so much that their effectiveness is put into question. Projecting these findings out to 6 months, on average 60% of stockings (flat or round knitted) do not exert effective therapeutic pressure after 6 months' regular wear. The measurement results lead to the conclusion that proper therapeutic care can only be achieved if a set of two regularly worn class 2 compression stockings is renewed twice a year.

Results for class 3 stockings are better.

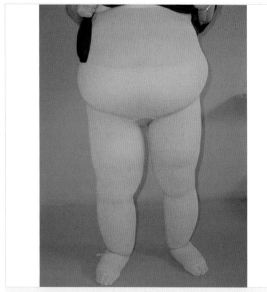

Fig. 13.21 Knee stockings and toecaps with Capri pants.

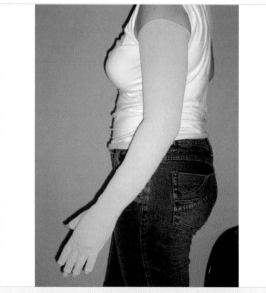

Fig. 13.23 Arm stocking and glove.

A choice is available between custom-fitted round- and flat-knitted stockings of different compression classes, and ready-made stockings of both types.

Difference between Flat-Knitted and Round-Knitted Stockings

Round-knitted: Round-knitted stockings are made on knitting needles arranged in a knitting cylinder. The result is a seamless knitted tube. The number of knitting needles in the cylinder is always the same and therefore the number of knitted stitches in a row is also the same. Hence, there are the same numbers of stitches around the narrow parts (foot, ankle, or wrist) as around the widest parts (thigh or upper arm). Varying widths are created through more or less prestretching of the thread.

Flat-knitted: Flat-knitted work pieces are made on straight rows of needles and only take on a stocking

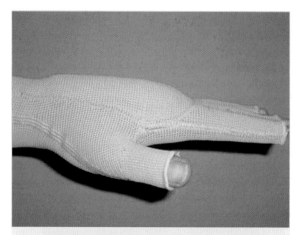

Fig. 13.22 Glove with reinforcement on the back of the hand.

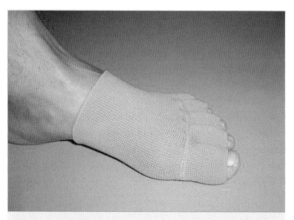

Fig. 13.24 Toecap.

Table 13.1 Overview of stockings with compression effect

Type	Compression class	Pressure and effect	Indication arm	Indication leg
Antiembolism stockings	N/A	Up to 17 mm Hg Very light	N/A	Only suitable for thrombosis and embolism prophylaxis in immobilized patients
Compression stockings	1	18–21 mm Hg Light superficial effect	Arm lymphedema	Slight varicosis without marked edema formation, incipient varicosis of pregnancy
	2	25.32 mm Hg Medium superficial effect	Arm lymphedema	Pronounced varicosis with edema formation, posttraumatic swelling after thrombophlebitis, obliteration, stripping, pronounced pregnancy varicosis, slight, incipient lymphedema
	3	36–46 mm Hg Strong superficial and depth effect	Arm lymphedema	Chronic venous insufficiency, severe edema tendency, secondary varicosis, atrophy blanche, after severe ulceration, lymphedema
	4	More than 59 mm Hg Enhanced depth effect	N/A	Lymphedema

shape when they are sewn together. The number of stitches can be varied depending on the edema. This ensures individual fitting and optimal pressure along the entire stocking even in cases of severe edema. Lymphedema is usually treated with flat-knitted products.

Compression strength and knitting type depend on the following criteria:
- What body part needs to be compressed?
- What type of lymphedema is being treated?
- What stage is the lymphedema?
- Does the edematous area show skin changes?
- Lipedema?
- Are there concomitant disorders (e.g., arthritis)?
- Age?
- Occupation?

During the maintenance phase of CDT, usually flat-knitted custom-fitted compression stockings are used. At the end of successful edema reduction treatment, and after consultation with the treating physician, a trained therapist or medical supplier will take measurements for the right fitting. Measurements must not be taken too soon, because the compression stocking cannot have the desired therapeutic effect until the extremity has been adequately decongested.

13.4 Therapeutic Exercises and Respiratory Therapy

13.4.1 Therapeutic Exercises

The principles are as follows:
- Muscle and joint movements increase passive lymph transport in the intramuscular, intracapsular, and intraligamentary lymph collectors.
- Muscle activity raises the heart rate. A raised heart rate raises the rate of arterial pulsation, which in turn increases lymphangiomotoricity, since the deep lymph vessels are always accompanied by arteries and every arterial pulsation is a stretch stimulus for the neighboring lymphangions.
- Carefully targeted exercises improve joint functions and the rheological properties of blood; that is, erythrocytes and leukocytes become more elastic and the blood plasma becomes thinner, which allows more erythrocytes to pass the blood capillaries per unit of time, and more O_2 reaches the tissue cells through the interstitium.
- Exercising also affects the breathing pattern. The increased inhalation and exhalation alter the intrathoracic pressure, which influences the lymph flow into the right and left venous angles. This altered breathing pattern accelerates the flow of lymph into the right and left venous angles.
- Special breathing techniques, such as abdominal breathing, lead to an increase in lymph movement, because the cisterna chyli and the lumen of the abdominal part of the thoracic duct passively contract and expand. With maximum inhalation, thoracic pressure drops and the thoracic part of the thoracic duct expands. Lymph is thus drawn out of the abdomen. On exhalation, the thoracic pressure returns to normal and the thoracic duct contracts. This causes passive transport of lymph to the venous angle. At the same time, the two subclavian veins expand and contract. A suction effect develops where the thoracic duct and the right intercostal trunk join (water-jet pump), that is, more lymph is sucked in by the venous system.

Lymphedema of the Arm

To reinforce the effects of the exercises, patients with arm lymphedema should only perform a daily exercise program when they are wearing bandages or a compression stocking. The exercises should be simple and easy to follow, and should not contain any swinging arm movements. In our experience, patients will perform a few well-chosen exercises and perform them as instructed. No more than three to five different exercises at home are required, repeated several times, to achieve the effect described earlier. If too many exercises are shown, the patients will not do any of them.

Arm movements in the form of proprioceptive neuromuscular facilitation (PNF) patterns or Brunkow's bracing exercises, with the instruction to work against an imaginary resistance, create intense muscular activity.

During the demonstration and practicing of the exercises, it often emerges that patients are having difficulty "imagining" resistance. In such cases, real resistance may be used during the learning phase in the form of therabands, which the patient may then take home. Carefully targeted resistance provided by the therapist also has a high educational effect on the patient during the learning phase. Equipment used in medical training therapy can also be used to support "imagined" resistance. Visualizations, such as "push the large rock to the side with your hand" or "lift the large rock to your left hip with your right hand," and so on, can also produce the desired muscular activity.

There is no limit to the creativity of the therapist. In specialized lymphology practices or in clinics providing inpatient treatment, group exercises are also an option. Patients are visibly more motivated in group exercises than when they have to exercise at home on their own.

Actual joint-specific limited mobility in any of the large joints of the extremities must be corrected using specific joint techniques. This can only be done in individual therapy sessions and requires knowledge of the biomechanics of the affected joints and training in manual therapy. Exercises invented by the patient or nonspecific exercises can make the impairment worse.

Muscular imbalances, faulty postures, and misalignments in the musculoskeletal system should be recognized and documented during the initial examination. Particularly in the case of unilateral arm lymphedema, the musculoskeletal system is almost bound to be subject to imbalances between the individual muscle groups, which cause faulty posture and misalignments. The lymph therapist must assess whether these musculoskeletal imbalances are constraining the lymphatic return. If a condition of the musculoskeletal system is found that impedes the lymph flow, this condition must be treated in parallel with the lymphedema treatment.

For inpatients at the Wittlinger Therapy Center, this means interdisciplinary collaboration between the massage therapist and the physical therapist during the decongestion phase.

In an outpatient decongestion phase, the practitioner (massage therapist or physical therapist) should encourage an interdisciplinary approach. It is also possible to design a patient's treatment plan in such a way that the physical therapy achieves meaningful, targeted, successful treatment of the lymphedema and of the diagnosed movement restriction.

Very good athletic activities for patients with arm lymphedema are swimming, Nordic walking, cross-country skiing, or walking with a walking stick in the hand of the affected extremity. So are working out with free weights and light training with exercise machines. The even, rhythmic movements of these types of sports lead to the same results as the exercise program given by the therapist.

Lymphedema of the Leg

Top priority for a meaningful program of therapeutic exercises aiming to promote lymphatic return is to wear bandages or compression stockings on the affected leg.

Here too, it is possible to think up a multitude of effective exercises, but this is often unnecessary because mobile patients usually do enough in their day-to-day life to encourage lymphatic return. Question the patients about the pattern of their movements at work, at home, and elsewhere. Is it enough, or are they sitting or lying down all day? If the latter, the leg lymphedema patient needs a therapeutic exercise plan. For example, he or she should walk a given distance every day, or climb a given number of stairs, or spend a given amount of time on the exercise bicycle.

These daily exertions are enough to achieve or maintain optimum treatment results with regard to the lymphatic reflux.

As in patients with arm edema, if examination has revealed disturbances in the musculoskeletal system, they must be treated with targeted joint and muscle techniques. Patients with unilateral leg lymphedema in particular complain about effects on gait, the spine, and the resulting additional symptoms that are caused. Targeted physiotherapeutic techniques from manual therapy, gait training, stretching, and the like improve the movement impairments. Over the course of treatment, a balance must be maintained between edema treatment and physiotherapy techniques.

Useful athletic activities are slow jogging, Nordic walking, hiking, swimming, bicycling, mountain biking, and of course exercise machine training in accordance with the prescribed training therapy.

13.4.2 Respiratory Therapy

Our inpatient clinic does not offer therapy sessions for respiration alone during the decongestion phase. Instead, respiratory therapy is integrated into the lymphedema patient's individual therapy sessions. If indicated, deep abdominal drainage, as described in the practice section, is part of this treatment. Another respiratory therapeutic procedure is the "half-moon position," a specific positioning technique with lateral trunk flexion and shoulder elevation. With the patient in this position, manual lymph drainage is performed. All the various other respiration-stimulating exercises available during inpatient care at the Wittlinger Therapy Center are offered in meditative group sessions.

13.4.3 Meditative Aspects

During the inpatient decongestion phase, we offer our lymphedema patients various classes and group therapies to help them learn to deal better with stress situations in their daily life. Our experience shows that everyday stress usually makes lymphedema worse. The aim of the meditative group therapies is to help patients find their own way of reducing stress factors as quickly as possible.

Autogenic training, yoga, Feldenkrais, Tai Chi, Qigong, and others can be of great help to patients.

13.5 Lymph Taping

Kinesio taping was developed in the 1970s by the Japanese physician Kase and was brought to the United States in the 1980s. Today numerous suppliers offer variations of the tape worldwide.

Below we will give you a brief introduction to lymph taping, which is not intended to be exhaustive. Several-day courses cover this topic in depth.

In this method, the tape creates a sort of "negative" pressure in the tissue underneath, leading to the following effects:

- Improved muscle function due to altered tension with an impact on muscle coordination.
- Decrease or elimination of circulatory restrictions, which is of particular interest in combination with

lymph drainage. In this way, a 24-hour effect can be provided.
- Activation of the endogenous analgesic system. Stimulation of mechanoreceptors activates the body's pain control system (gate control theory of pain).
- Improved joint function. Stimulation of joint receptors activates the muscles, producing greater stability; proprioception is improved, and stimulus response is faster.

We regard lymph taping as useful support to manual lymph drainage/CDT, especially in areas (thorax, face) that are difficult to bandage.

13.5.1 Lymph Tape

The tape is modeled on the strength and thickness of the skin, and in this it differs from other tapes. The basic substance is a cotton fabric containing cotton-wrapped latex-free stretch fibers. It can be stretched lengthwise, with an elasticity of approximately 140%. The material is waterproof, but air and moisture permeable, allowing moisture to be released to the outside. A special thermo-active adhesive made of acrylic is applied in a wavelike pattern to the tape.

The skin-friendly tape is applied for 5 to 7 days (no longer) and leaves nothing behind when removed. It can be combined with other therapies, such as essential oils or magnetic field treatment.

Lymph Tape and Lymph Stasis

Lymph tape is indicated for various malfunctions of the musculoskeletal system and for lymph stasis. When applying the tape, the therapist focuses on the regional lymph nodes while heeding the watersheds. This special application technique—via pressure and pull as well as through regular body movements—enables loosening of the connective tissue followed by stimulating lymphangiomotoricity. Because tissue pressure directly under the tape is reduced, the volume is also reduced and pain recedes.

The lymph taping itself can be done as a fan shape, I-strip, or spiral strip (▶ **Fig. 13.25**).

The majority of contraindications are the same as for regular taping, that is, malignant disease, acute inflammation (e.g., erysipelas/cellulitis), acute deep vein thrombosis, superficial phlebitis and thrombosis, acute allergic contact eczema, and severe (untreated) cardiac insufficiency.

How to Use Lymph Tape in Lymphology (This Example Assumes a Patient with Arm Edema)

Ensure that the skin is dry and free from oil. To improve wear comfort and avoid skin irritation, body hair in the area of application must be removed. This also considerably improves the adhesion of the tape.

Tape measurements are taken directly on the patient (▶ **Fig. 13.26**). Cut the tape according to the measurements; cut the tape into thirds and round off all the corners (▶ **Fig.13.27**). Remove the paper from the anchor of the tape and place the anchor on the patient's skin without prestretching the tape or prepositioning the patient for taping (▶ **Fig. 13.28**). The anchor must be placed well within the lymph area into which you want the lymph-obligatory load to drain. The individual strips are then applied with the patient maximally prepositioned for taping (but without stretching the tape). This means having the patient in spinal extension for the application of anterior strips, and in lateral flexion for the application of lateral strips. The patient's taping position is enhanced by elevating the arm (▶ **Figs. 13.29** and ▶ **Fig. 13.30**). Depending on the elasticity of the patient's skin, skin folds result in the neutral-zero position, which is an indication of the effectiveness of the tape (▶ **Fig. 13.31**). After a maximum of 7 days, the tape is removed and disposed of.

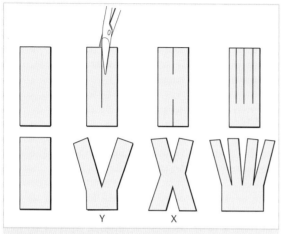

Fig. 13.25 Taping shapes: fan shape, I-strip/spiral strip.

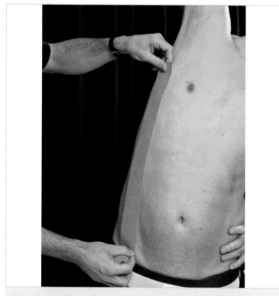

Fig. 13.26 Taking the tape measurements directly on the patient.

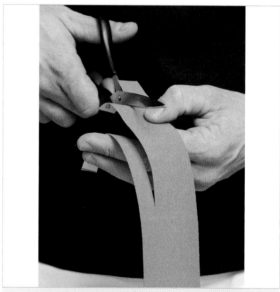

Fig. 13.27 Cutting the tape for a W shape.

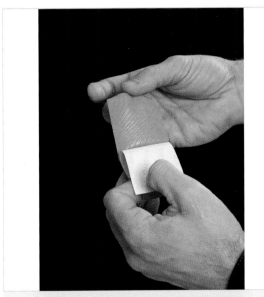

Fig. 13.28 Pulling the paper off the tape for anchoring.

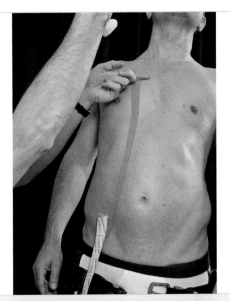

Fig. 13.29 Applying the tape with the patient maximally prepositioned for taping (here: extension)

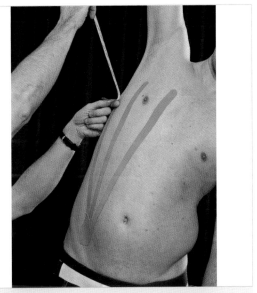

Fig. 13.30 Application of the lateral strip, without stretching the tape, but with the patient in the taping position.

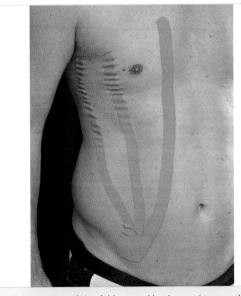

Fig. 13.31 Typical skin folds caused by the tape's own pull toward the anchor.

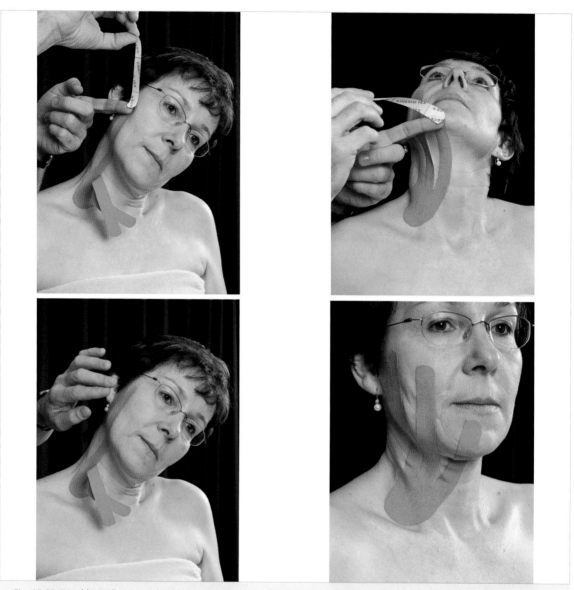

Fig. 13.32 Possible application technique in a patient with unilateral facial lymphedema in whom the terminus was not radiated.

13.6 Further Information

13.6.1 Useful Addresses

- **American Lymphedema Framework Project**
  https://www.facebook.com/
  AmericanLymphedemaFrameworkProject

- **Canadian Lymphedema Framework**
  4800 Dundas Street W, Suite 204
  Toronto, Ontario M9A 1B1
  Canada
  Phone: +1 647-693-1083
  Email: admin@canadalymph.ca
  http://canadalymph.ca/
  https://de-de.facebook.com/canadalymph/

- **International Society of Lymphology**
  http://www.u.arizona.edu/~witte/ISL.htm

- **Healthy Steps, Inc.**
  http://www.gohealthysteps.com/
  https://www.facebook.com/
  Healthy-Steps-111374642239329/

- **Lymphatic Education & Research Network**
  261 Madison Avenue, 9th Floor
  New York, NY 10016
  Phone: (516) 625-9675
  Fax: (516) 625-9410
  Email: lern@lymphaticnetwork.org
  http://lymphaticnetwork.org/
  https://www.facebook.com/LymphaticResearch

- **Lymphedema Association of Ontario**
  101-330 Bronte St. South
  Milton, ON L9T 7X1
  Canada
  Email: info@lymphontario.ca
  https://www.facebook.com/pages/Lymphedema-
  Association-of-Ontario/114492005247973

- **McGill Lymphedema Research Program
  University Health Centre (MUHC)**
  5252 Blvd. de Maisonneuve West, 105b
  Montreal, Quebec
  H4A 3S5
  Phone: 514-934-1934 ext. 78716
  https://www.mcgill.ca/lymphedema-research/

- **North American Vodder Association (NAVALT)**
  https://navalt.wordpress.com

Part V

Historical Background

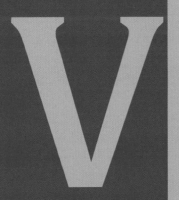

14 Historical Background

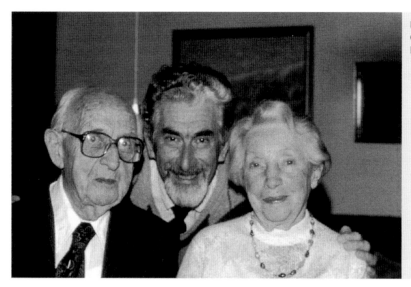

Dr. Emil Vodder † 1986
Günther Wittlinger † 1986
Estrid Vodder † 1996

This photograph was taken in 1984 at the presentation of the Rohrbach medal to Dr. Vodder by the German Association of Physical Therapy (VPT). The VPT had thus honored a man who left us all an excellent and effective massage method. Dr. Emil Vodder and his wife, Estrid, devoted their lives to manual lymph drainage and its dissemination. They called upon Günther Wittlinger to act as defender and advocate of manual lymph drainage.

14.1 Preface to the First Edition 1978

The following preface was written by Dr. Emil Vodder, creator of the manual lymph drainage method.

Although my wife and I completed the elaboration of the method in France during the years 1932–1936, we were unable to write a book about it until 40 years later. We have been travelling around Europe for many years now, holding lectures and courses to explain the structure and function of the lymph system by means of drawings and manuals. Needless to say, the scientific world was not yet ready for our findings and would not accept our hypothesis and empirical evidence. The lymph system was an unknown factor in the field of physical therapy, an unexplored and dangerous *no-man's-land*. It was considered inadvisable to massage the lymphatic nodes, since it was thought that the treatment would spread bacteria and viruses. Children with swollen nodes in the neck, for example, were said to have *scrofulosis* and were operated on to remove the affected nodes. Appendicitis and spleen operations were also carried out without considering that, in so doing, the

defense mechanisms of the body could be impaired—a hypothesis that later research proved to be true. Doctors in Ancient Greece knew about the lymph system in the intestines, that is, the chylous vessels, which resemble white chains of pearls and contain the milky-white chylous sap. Herophilus wrote that "vessels emerging from the intestines enter a number of gland-like bodies and not the portal vein." These gland-like bodies are our lymph nodes. In the Middle Ages anatomical research was regarded as sinful; scientific discoveries were therefore few during this period. In the Renaissance, however, a large number of important findings emerged. Many schools of anatomy were established, for example in Salerno, Bologna, Padua, Montpellier, Paris, Leyden, Copenhagen, and Uppsala. In 1662, in Padua an Italian by the name of Aselli displayed the lymph vessels in a dog's intestines. He called them *chyliferi*—shimmering milky-white veins. Six years later in London William Harvey published his exciting discovery, namely that the blood makes a complete circuit in the body. Two students, Jean Pecquet in Montpellier (1647) and Olaf Rudbeck in Sweden, discovered the thoracic duct in dogs. Rudbeck was a Renaissance genius who founded the still existing *Theatrum Anatomicum* in Uppsala. In 1653 he published *Nova exercitatio anatomica* and called the newly discovered vessels vasa serosa and the lymph nodes *glandulae aquosae*. As a favorite of Queen Christina of Sweden, he had the honor of demonstrating his anatomical findings to the royal court. In July 1637 a young Dane, Thomas Bartholin, was studying at the University of Leyden in Holland. His scientific research was facilitated by the existence of the *Theatrum Anatomicum* in Leyden, a library, a botanical garden, and a hospital overflowing with patients.

Up to that time only "lunatic asylums" and hospitals for plague victims had been built in Northern Europe. Bartholin studied Aselli's lymph vessels and learned how to inject gum resin and indigo into the vessels to render them visible. Over a period of 10 years he visited many countries, studying languages and natural sciences. When he finally returned to Denmark he had become a renowned scientist and took over the newly built *Theatrum Anatomicum* in Copenhagen. He was the first to describe the entire lymph system. He wrote four papers in Latin, dedicated to King Frederick III, describing the lymph system as a natural process that purifies the body and regulates irritation, swelling, and edema. In *Vasa lymphatica*, 1652–1654, he describes his findings on lymph vessels and nodes in humans. No researcher had as yet used any special term for the lymph fluid. Bartholin called the vessels *vasa lymphatica* and their content lymph—clear water, from the Latin *limpidus*, meaning clear. Twenty years later in Schaffhausen, Johan Conrad Peyer described the intestinal lymph aggregations now called Peyer's patches. Research was continued in many countries during the following centuries. However, lymphology, the science of lymph and tissue fluids, was not developed until recently. The water content of the body should be studied as a whole because all organs and organic systems are intimately connected. The ground substance is ubiquitous in the body, although it varies according to its environment, as described by Professor Hugo Grau in Dr. Zilch's instructive work, *Lymph System and Lymphatismus*. This book is highly recommended to all students interested in lymph research and immunology (Munich, 1963). Very early in our studies we were of the conviction that the human body should be regarded as a whole. We were inspired by the writings of Claude Bernard, Alexis Carrel, and Cecil Drinker, who convinced us of the importance of the omnipresent lymph system in the body. Alexis Carrel, the father of modern organ transplants, confirmed this view when he received the Nobel Prize in 1912 for his research on the cultivation of living cells. This was an exciting period, since we foresaw what the future held for us. Carrel's classic experiment proved that the cells in a chicken's heart stayed alive if the lymph fluid was continuously renewed. Later we based our method of lymphatic regeneration of the skin on this principle. We were certain that the lymph fluid was the source of miraculous hidden forces. But despite great strides made in the field of biology, the lymphocytes retained their secret until in the middle of this century it was discovered that the nuclei of the lymphocytes contain the life-giving substance deoxyribonucleic acid (DNA), which is the prime substance of life and the vehicle of genetic traits in all organisms. Research on the lymph system reached its peak when immunologists established that lymphocytes produce antibodies to protect the body against viruses and infections. It is of interest to note that 30 years ago one of the first lymph researchers in the United States, Professor Cecil Drinker, prophesied that the lymph system would be recognized as the most important organic system in humans and animals. We lived 11 years of our youth in the inspiring atmosphere of France—5 years on the sunny Riviera and 6 busy years in Paris. By studying everything that we could find about lymph and by putting what we learned into practice we were able to develop hypotheses which have long since been confirmed by researchers. One day a client came to our physical therapy institute in Cannes for treatment of a nose and throat infection, migraine and blemished, oily skin. As usual, I closed my eyes while I palpated the hard, swollen, cervical lymph nodes. I suddenly imagined a nasal sinus covered with shimmering lymph vessels. In my mind I also saw their drainage focused in the neck, the lymph node chains that act as a natural draining system for the skin, mucosa, and meninges, that is, for all the organs and nodes in the head and neck. As far as I know, this complex had never previously been interpreted as a natural drainage apparatus for the entire head region. I asked myself whether obstruction in the severely swollen lymph nodes could be the underlying cause of these different ailments. Were the impurities of the skin and the catarrh of the mucous membranes the result of the malfunction of the lymph nodes? Would it be possible to unblock the drainage system by treatment with appropriate massage techniques? Had I just discovered a universal therapy to cure the lymphatic syndrome? This hypothesis has since been substantiated a thousand times over by such treatment, which has no side effects whatsoever. My patient was completely cured of all his ailments after ten facial massages using gentle rotary pumping movements over the lymph node chains. Nor did the ailments recur. Did the lymph have undreamt-of healing powers? No doubt! In 1933 we moved to Paris where we continued our research, especially with regard to the anatomical and physiological aspects of the lymph vessel system. Professor Rouvière had just published his book *L'Anatomie des Lymphatiques de l'Homme* ("Anatomy of the lymphatic vessels in man"). Alexis Carrel had written an invaluable book called *Der Mensch—das unbekannte Wesen* ("Man—the unknown"), and most important was the huge atlas by the anatomist Phil. Sappey, which contained a collection of very beautiful copperplate engravings that we used a great deal during our course in Manual Lymph Drainage. (Phil. Sappey: *Description et iconographie des vaisseaux lymphatiques considérés chez l'homme et les vertébrés*, Paris 1885—"Description and iconography of the lymph vessels in man and the vertebrates.") In 1936 we succeeded in compiling a simple systematic list of massage movements, using our intuition and extensive practical experience. An entirely new set of massage techniques was necessary. There had to be circular pumping and draining movements with a pressure of less than 30 mm Hg (now called torr) so as to *prevent* blood filling. We employed gentle stationary circles on the lymph nodes, an area that no one had previously dared to massage, palpating with the tips or the entire length of the fingers. Massaging was always in the direction of the clavicular fossa, the terminus of all lymph pathways in the body. The method was conceived not only for facial treatment, that is, for cosmetic and preventive measures, but also to cure illnesses. Our therapeutic treatment often produced surprising and rapid results. Positive effects were always obtained if *correct, slow and rhythmic movements* were employed, whether we were treating the patient for skin rejuvenation, hematomas caused by accidents, eczema, varicose veins, or ulcerous legs. This was of course the fundamental principle: we were stimulating the lymph flow. It was now time to present our findings to the public. An important exhibition took place in Paris in the spring of 1936 with a theme which particularly attracted me: "Santé et Beauté" ("Health and Beauty"). It was a great success, and the newspapers reported on "lymph drainage—a revolutionary skin treatment." I had written an article in French which appeared in the Parisian journal *Santé pour Tous* ("Health for everyone") for which I was coeditor. It was later translated into Danish and Swedish (see page 135). After spending 11 instructive years in France; we were forced to return to our home town of Copenhagen at the outbreak of the Second World War. We began again and founded a new manual lymph drainage institute which we have now been running for 25 years. As we had already called the new field *lymphology*, we called the students that we trained *lymph therapists*. But it was not until the 1950s that other countries showed any interest in our work. Then we were invited to give lectures and courses in various countries, which we have now been doing for the last 20 years. We have personally trained thousands of students from Europe. We also employ assistants and a full-time staff who continue to teach our original method and life's work—"Dr. Vodder's Manual Lymph Drainage." What progress has science made in the last decade? Modern developments such as electron microscopy, tracer methods, computers, and macromolecular chemistry have also provided new insight into aspects of the lymph system for which no logical explanation had been offered until then. For example, researchers discovered the vital substance DNA in the lymphocyte nucleus, which forms the very basis of life and is the vehicle of genetic traits in all cells. It contains the blueprints for all the tissues of our body, as already programmed in the fetus. A healthy lymph system promotes healthy body tissues and body functions. The lymph system is not only the source of good health, it also guards against infection. Research on the lymph system, formerly known as *the neglected child of medicine*, reached its summit recently with elucidation of the immune system. Renowned lymphologists and immunologists have proved that the lymphocytes are responsible

for the production of antibodies to combat viruses and infections ranging from influenza to cancer. At the very beginning of our research my wife and I interpreted the body as a whole and thus regarded the lymph system as a source of life. The lymph system that originally developed from the primordial soup is universal and combines the macrocosm and microcosm within us. It represents the omnipresent living environment of the body because all nutrients and vital substances must flow throughout the lymph interspaces by way of a *transit stretch* to the cells. The term "lymph" has taken on a broad meaning in modern lymph therapy. As far as our technique is concerned it covers not only the interstitial lymph that carries the nutrient fluid to the cells but also indirectly the fluid circulating in the protoplasm of trillions of cells. It should be noted that some lymphologists insist that the connective tissue fluid is not the same as the lymph fluid. On the other hand, it is said that the lymph fluid develops in the connective tissue. One thing, however, is certain: the lymph system not only serves to clean tissues through drainage, but is also a protection and defense mechanism and carries out vital functions. Just as the red blood corpuscles act as vehicles to transport oxygen and carbon dioxide, the lymph fluid carries the lymph-obligatory load (i.e., a mixture of vital substances and toxins) back to the blood stream. The lymph contains nearly all plasma-protein constituents necessary to the cells as building substances and nutrients as well as vitamins, hormones, and destroyed cells (waste products), for example, as a result of hematomas or other injuries. Since none of these large molecules can pass through the venous walls, their transport by the lymph system is essential to life. For this reason, it is clear that the lymphocytes carry building substances to the cell tissues and that effective use of manual lymph drainage can greatly accelerate the process of building new cells. Millions of lymphocytes are continuously being produced in the lymph tissues (in the palatine and pharyngeal tonsils, the spleen, the lymph nodules and Peyer's patches). Recent research findings show that an average of 35 billion lymphocytes enter the blood every day through the terminal ducts that empty into large veins in the lower part of the neck. This number can increase up to as much as 562 billion during periods of stress. Professor Collard of Brussels convincingly demonstrated the forward movement of lymph during manual lymph drainage treatment. He illustrated this by means of color film using a contrast medium. Classical massage techniques, on the other hand, had no drainage effect whatsoever. Professor Kuhnke's investigations led him to the same conclusions. He demonstrated that a pressure of 30 mm Hg was correct and also necessary to remove proteinaceous tissue swelling (edema). Research carried out by Casley-Smith in Australia showed that normal massage techniques are much too forceful to allow drainage in the interstitium and may hinder removal (lymph obstruction). The lymph system is even more fascinating as a defense mechanism in the immune system and represents the most promising research field for young investigators today. Many years ago, Professor Olliviéro, a renowned biologist in Paris, made the following humorous comparison: "Man," he said, "is an amphibian. Even the most beautiful feminine body is no more than an aquarium with 50 L of lukewarm seawater in which trillions of cells live and fight for survival." The unicellular organisms, which originated from the sea, have accumulated all essential chemical genetic substances on the endless road of evolution. In the aqueous environment the amoebas, or rather the lymphocytes, had to learn as unicellular organisms to protect the *private sphere.* They formed an outer covering or a membrane, so as not to be diluted or destroyed. The chemistry of life was thus protected in the fashion by the cellular membrane. Evolution as we know it could then begin. The existence of cells in the primordial ocean was naturally accompanied by the need for food. The cells that knew best how to exploit the energy resources flourished and gained supremacy over the less efficient cells. The best and purest source of nutrients was found in the cells themselves—harmful substances and toxins came from the exterior. Gradually some cells joined together—strength in numbers—and the inseparable cells survived. The chemical processes that take place in the body were the best and most ingenious that Mother Nature could have developed. These concern the substances that regulate metabolism, that is, sugar and fat that provide energy, amino acids that form proteins, and phospholipids that make up cellular membranes. Man has evolved unremittingly and has emerged the victor of a 3-billion-year fight for survival. However, the original struggle that began in the primordial ocean when the first cell turned against its own kind has never ceased despite culture, mercy, and altruism. Today we are living as always on a seabed of bacteria and viruses. The most vicious warriors measure only 7 microns in diameter and yet are our deadliest foes. These tiny enemies carry out silent lightning attacks. Viruses and bacteria that enter a cut finger or the mucous membrane can reach the brain cells seconds later. For this very reason our immune system maintains a huge arsenal of white blood corpuscles. A person weighing 70 kg has an average of 26 billion granulocytes and macrophages (phagocytes) from the bone marrow at the ready. In addition there are other groups of chemical *guards* and microbiological *killer cells.* Professor Gowans of Oxford stated in a lecture: "There is no doubt that part of our ability to survive in an environment full of hostile micro-organisms depends on the strength of our huge army of lymphocytes." As a preface to this first textbook I have written a retrospective report on the development of manual lymph drainage and have also provided an outline of scientific efforts aimed at

disclosing the all-important secrets of the lymph system. We express our deep gratitude to Mr. and Mrs. Wittlinger, the directors of the Dr. Vodder School in Walchsee, Tirol, for meeting a long-felt need with this textbook.

Copenhagen-Bagsvaerd, January 1978
Dr. phil. Emil Vodder

14.2 Lymph Drainage—A New Therapeutic Method Serving Cosmetic Care

First Publication about Dr. Vodder's Manual Lymph Drainage, an Original Work by Dr. Emil Vodder, Paris 1936.

14.2.1 The Beauty of the Face

A poet describes the eyes as the mirror of the soul. In modern body care, the face could be called the mirror of health. The face not only reflects our feelings, our good mood (or sorrow), our character; it also reveals our state of health, the balance or imbalance of mind and body. The face is also more exposed than the body to the elements (i.e., wind, rain, and temperature changes). The face *experiences* more than the body; it is "on show" more. Thus, in the morning, we notice the first signs of aging on our faces, long before the body itself ages. With this shock the never-ending attempt begins to maintain beauty and radiance. Therefore, it is not surprising that from time immemorial we have endeavored to improve and brighten up the appearance of the face. Neither is it surprising that women who see their youth disappearing spend their time and money on trying to halt this process. Do they succeed? That depends on how they invest their time and money. Unfortunately, there are many charlatans with bottomless pockets. Every day incredible sums of money are spent on worthless skin care and beauty products. What we should be clear about is that it is not enough for us to merely superficially conceal the inadequacies of our face, like a sick person who believes they can get rid of their health problems by taking pills. Likewise, simply applying a rejuvenating cream to sagging skin on the face is not enough. These days, most beauty care products are merely cosmetic. In other words, one cannot change the face with surface treatments: exfoliation and dermabrasion with chemical products, just like smoothing out wrinkles and tightening the skin with certain cosmetic products, is only a trick. The effect only lasts for a short time because the root of the problem has not been addressed.

14.2.2 Is Aging Unavoidable?

If the world is continually developing, why can't we also benefit from the advancements? Why is it that we cannot maintain perpetual youth? It is so nice to be young and supple, to radiate with beauty and a zest for life. Young and healthy people are simply successful in everything! Why therefore does nature allow us to age?

To find the answers we will embark on an investigative journey through the wondrous world of our bodies.

14.2.3 The Blood Vessel System

We begin our search in the heart itself, in a small vehicle that we will call white blood cells. We can examine life more closely in the individual factories along the channel formed by our blood vessel network. At first, we are surrounded by numerous smaller boats: the red blood cells which are loaded with oxygen, the fuel for all cell activity. The water in our current is called plasma and is yellow: it contains nutrients and waste. Each heartbeat sends our small vehicle, in the incredible time of 23 seconds, through the whole blood vessel system (arteries, capillaries, and veins) until it has reached the heart again.

14.2.4 The Lymph Vessel System

Generally, this system is not so well known, because when we speak of "circulation" we always refer to the blood circulation. A new system? Absolutely not; the lymph system is the origin of life. For the lymph is the nutrient liquid for the very first collection of cells, just as it is for that living palace of millions of cells: the complete human organism. However, this system was discovered relatively late: there are two noteworthy 17th century scholars of the lymph system: Pequet (1647), who discovered and named the cisterna chyli, and the Dane, Bartholin, who discovered the lymph vessel system 3 years later. Thus, we live in lymph, that is, our tissues are washed in lymph. It supplies us with the life-giving nutrients necessary for body development. If we continue on our journey, we see how youth, life, and death are dependent on lymph and its renewal. Our vehicle has now left the capillaries through a small secret door and, in this manner, we can distinguish between the two circulatory systems. Lymph is a whitish fluid. The flow in the lymph channels is sluggish and we glide calmly through because there is no pulsation here coming from the heart, driving us forward every few seconds. However, we still move forward with the help of a carefully thought-out valve system that prevents backflow: we pass thousands of filters until we reach the large lakes of the serous cavities. In this way, we can visit all the regions of the body from head to feet: the labyrinth of the ear, the membranes of the brain and spinal cord, the pleura, etc. We run into flooded regions (edema and infiltrations) and dry areas where life functions slower and cells degenerate because the lymph was the source of their renewal. The lymph vessel system therefore represents a type of sewage system, eliminating wastes produced by the working cells and carrying them to organs which get rid of them—the lymph nodes.

14.2.5 The Lymph Nodes

The lymph nodes are filters, whose function is to hold back and destroy the harmful substances, poisons, and bacteria. A lymph node consists of adenoid tissue and, like the spleen and tonsils, continually produces white blood cells. These cells defend the body against invasion and poisoning, and their activity is heightened during infectious diseases. So what happens in the lymph system during an infection (e.g., during a heavy cold)? We experience a battle. The body reacts to the invasion of bacteria in the nose with an immediate assembly of troops, a total security force. The mucous membranes swell up, the lymph vessels and nodes enlarge, the white blood cells destroy bacteria and take them away. Generally, the battle is finished in the lymph nodes, which can be compared to castles. It is fascinating to watch this process under the microscope and it gave rise to Claude Bernard's conclusion: "Bacteria themselves are not the decisive factor, solely the surrounding territory." We should be aware that a poorly functioning lymph circulation lowers our defense, which opens the door to every infection: catarrh, chronic colds, sinusitis, sore throat, angina, etc. Unfortunately, this condition of congestion, which can be traced back to a worsening stagnation of lymph, also has a detrimental effect on one's appearance. This is the deeper cause of a series of cosmetic flaws such as swelling, reddening, puffiness, bags under the eyes, pimples, couperose, etc. Stagnation of the lymph flow therefore has catastrophic results for health and beauty: the lymph circulation has to be stimulated again at all costs, and this is achieved with the help of manual lymph drainage. Manual lymph drainage cleanses the lymph, the swelling in the mucous membranes goes down, and consequently the cause of the problems is eradicated.

14.2.6 Natural Regeneration of the Skin through Lymph Drainage

Before we go back to the heart, we conclude our investigative journey by examining the skin. We see that the skin cells wear out and, thanks to a process called mitosis, are constantly replaced by young cells. We have seen how the necessary, life-sustaining nutrients leave the blood with the help of osmosis, pass into the lymph, and thus reach the cells. Assuming this exchange cannot take place, the lymph vessels become blocked with stagnant, old lymph: the blood flows, to no avail, past each little secret door and transports the nutrients to another location. This is how the body becomes poisoned by its own waste. During my research work in the laboratories of the faculty in Copenhagen (1922–1924), under the direction of the renowned cancer researcher Professor Fibiger, the significance of the cell environment in lymph circulation for living, diseased, and dead cells was suddenly clear to me. I understood clearly how the perpetual youth of the cell depends on this fluid (the lymph). Dr. Carrel's experiments have supported my theories. He was able to keep embryonic cells alive for over 10 years, whereas the normal life expectancy is only 4–5 years. This was possible thanks to the lymphatic milieu which was changed every 2 days. Conclusion: If the milieu and cell activity stagnate then the cells will degenerate, age, and die. If the milieu is constantly renewed, then life flourishes and the cells divide. Then the wrinkled and tired skin can regenerate itself, it becomes fresh and elastic, and the tired worn-out appearance in the face disappears. A real metamorphosis is experienced, a natural regeneration that comes from within. Our new therapeutic method is therefore based on these facts.

14.2.7 Lymph Drainage

After many years of clinical experience and research, a rational method of treatment has been successfully developed which enables renewal of the lymph, activation of the circulation, stimulation of cell activity, and regeneration of the facial tissue. Lymph drainage is a healthy, natural, painless, and absolutely effective method which gives a new basis to life, health, and beauty.

Original translation from French into German by Mechtild Yvon, MA. Phil., Vienna. We thank Mrs. Banniza of Menden for her great effort in procuring this article. Nothing has been added to this article. The special thing about it is that it was written 74 years ago. Vodder's ideas of that time were proved correct through diverse experiments. His manual techniques need no improvement or further development. The method requires only further research into its sphere of influence. This is the task before us today and, at the same time, a legacy left to us.

Note

At the time this article was written, all bodily fluid excepting blood and cellular fluid was described as lymph. Now this is referred to in the nomenclature as connective-tissue fluid, or interstitial fluid. Only the fluid in the lymph vessel is nowadays called "lymph."

14.3 Emil Vodder—His Life and Manual Lymph Drainage

While studying my records I realized how difficult it is to describe a person's life. On the one hand there is the curriculum vitae filled with facts, and on the other hand there is the person who creates these facts, the consequences of which shape his life. A multitude of views exists about our doings, the path we follow or are led to, and what we make of it all. Therefore, I will begin with the facts and try to weave in the actual life that was lived. Emil Vodder was born on February 20, 1896 in Copenhagen. After finishing school, he studied drawing and art history as well as comparative linguistics, including 10 languages. He then worked at the Copenhagen Royal Danish Nautical Charts Archive for 6 years. As a hobby, he studied voice and cello. At the University of Copenhagen he enrolled in biology, mineralogy, and botany, as well as in medicine, cytology, and microscopy. Very early on he was interested in physical medicine. He fell ill with malaria and had to suspend his studies in the eighth semester. Later, he was not readmitted to complete his studies. In 1928 he received his PhD from the University of Brussels with a dissertation in art history. In 1929, he and his wife Estrid, a naturopath, moved to the French Riviera. In Cannes he founded an institute for physical therapy, where he began treating patients. Early on, Vodder had an interest in the lymphatic system and its exploration. Interestingly, Vodder was acquainted with the works of scientists who had in one way or another done research into the mysterious "clear water" centuries earlier. Brief references to almost all their names and research work can be found in his preface to the first edition. Due to his studies in relevant literature, Vodder was convinced from the beginning that the human being is a biological unit. Through his study of writings by Bernard, Carrel, and Drinker he realized that lymph is an omnipresent living environment. In his preface to the first edition of our book, published in 1978, Vodder quoted Drinker's prophecy:

"The lymphatic system is the most important organ system in the life of humans and animals." At this point I must mention a comment from Professor Weissleder: "We must assume that the majority of diseases develop through micro-edema in the connective tissue." To underpin the concordance of these two statements, I should like to add that in Drinker's and Vodder's times, the fluid part of the connective tissue was called "lymph." It is easy to see that if micro-edema changes the "lymph"—that is, connective tissue—which is the living environment, this may be the basis of many diseases. But back now to the year 1929, when Vodder was working with patients, gathering experience, and constructing hypotheses that were daring at the time. He palpated swollen lymph nodes in the neck of patients suffering from skin blemishes, migraines, and sinusitis. He had the vision that congestion in the lymph glands (today called nodes) was the underlying cause of these various disorders. The lymph nodes had become unable to fulfill their task of cleansing the tissue. He pondered whether it would be possible to release the congestion through a suitable massage technique, like opening the sluices in a dam, so that the surplus would drain off and everything would return to normal. Carefully circling the skin with a pumping motion achieved the result he had envisaged. The pioneering act—and some might call it imprudence—was to treat the swollen cervical lymph nodes even though at the time merely touching them was absolutely taboo. The symptoms disappeared and he asked himself if he had found a successful universal therapy for lymphatic syndrome. The Vodders continued their biological studies in Paris. In particular, they devoted themselves to the anatomy and physiology of the lymphatic vascular system. In a large atlas, Vodder found a collection of very beautiful copperplate prints by the anatomist Sappey (*Description et iconographie des vaisseaux lymphatiques considérés chez l'homme et les vertébrés*, Paris 1885). These copperplate prints were essentially the foundation of Emil Vodder's systematic and precise working method, which he developed through a combination of intuition and giving many treatments. An entirely new massage technique was necessary, which he performed with pumping circular movements and very light pressure, in order to avoid at all costs hyperemia. Earlier scientists including Winiwarter had described the treatment of edema and realized that light pressure and bandaging are helpful. But it is Vodder's achievement to have given us a technique, with its very subtle manipulations, that allows us as therapists to treat individual disorders in a targeted way and perform an infinite amount of good. At the outbreak of World War II, the Vodders had to return to Copenhagen. A new beginning under difficult circumstances lay before them. In the early 1960s, Mrs. Bartetzko and Dr. Asdonk came into contact with Vodder and became interested in his method. Therapists today owe a great deal to Dr. Asdonk. As a physician he recognized the enormous importance of this method and put together the first list of indications for us. Lymphedema as we know it today was not on the list. In 1966, the first contact was made between Günther Wittlinger and Dr. Vodder. In 1967, Vodder, Asdonk, and Wittlinger founded the Society for Dr. Vodder's Manual Lymph Drainage. The first congress took place that year and was a great success. The problem in those days was that no physician or scientist could imagine that a manual technique could have a beneficial effect on the lymphatic system. Sadly, this problem still exists today, especially abroad. Vodder himself once said: "I discovered this method too soon. Nobody understands me." A landmark in the acquisition of evidence of the decongesting effect of manual lymph drainage was the statement by Professor Mislin that the particular technique employed in Dr. Vodder's Manual Lymph Drainage, using light circular motions to move the skin, and with pressure that increases and decreases, stimulates the lymph vessels—or, rather, the lymphangions—of the skin to increased contractions. As Vodder said time and again, if the source of lymph is the connective tissue, this would substantiate the claim that this method could decongest the connective tissue, remove micro-edema in the connective tissue of the skin, and eradicate the source of many evils. In the 1970s, Mislin said: "If Vodder had not created his method in the way he did, we would have to invent it immediately." As mentioned before, Emil Vodder viewed the human being as a unit. If one part is sick, the whole person is sick. That was his proposition. Describing his personality is very difficult. I consider him an extraordinary human being. The method he created is simple but brilliant, difficult to learn, but unique in its effect. In addition to all the therapeutic effects, the delicate circular motion, always attending to the needs of the tissue, gives the patient a very pleasant sensation. This was damaging for the method at first, as people claimed we were just stroking the patient. Lymph drainage therapists do not like hearing this. The method was derided as quackery. This was a harsh word to those who had used it with much success. In the end it was scientists, and the trials they conducted confirming the effectiveness of the method, that helped Vodder's lymph drainage to achieve the breakthrough. That was also the beginning of lymphedema therapy. The method was finally accepted by the German statutory health insurance system, and in the 25 years since this acceptance, it has become the most frequently prescribed form of massage. It must be reiterated that only a massage pressure that is adapted to the tissue being treated—it may range from very light to quite heavy—will produce the desired result. With the addition of bandaging, which turned out to be hugely effective, contemporary conservative lymphedema therapy was born. A combination of various therapies could now be employed to improve the lymphedema patient's wellbeing and quality of life. Vodder was a witty and modest person. His knowledge was comprehensive—and not just with regard to lymph. He also concerned himself extensively with immunology, and here he found confirmation of the theory he had held since the early 1930s, that lymph nodes also have an immunological function, and as part of the lymphatic system play an important role in immunology. In our many encounters, which despite some lively debates were very harmonious, my husband and I came to know Emil Vodder as an erudite man, always open to discussion. He taught us a great deal and set us an example in the way he lived. His words were our incentive: "The greatest goal of our lives must be to find our path, recognize it, and follow it consistently." Emil Vodder lived his own life accordingly, and Günther Wittlinger became the fellow campaigner who ensured the survival of the method in its original form. Emil Vodder was frequently challenged to sell his method and get rich. He withstood those challenges with a little smile, saying: "I do not sell my life." In 1984, the Association of Physical Therapy awarded him the Rohrbach medal for his lifetime achievement. This medal was accompanied by the recognition of a professional association that Emil Vodder was the creator of the eponymous *Dr. Vodder's Manual Lymph Drainage*. Vodder died in Copenhagen in February 1986, shortly before his 90th birthday. His wife Estrid was faithfully at his side during all these years, assisting him in his workshops, and accompanying him on many lecture tours. She died 10 years after him, shortly before her 100th birthday. Their son Arne, a noted interior architect, lives in Copenhagen with his family. There must be few human beings who have had such a lasting effect on physical therapy and enriched it in the way Emil Vodder did. Many scientists, physicians, and therapists have contributed to the acceptance and recognition in medicine and physiotherapy of the method of manual lymph drainage that he created more than 70 years ago.

Lecture given on the occasion of the 75th birthday of Prof. Dr. Horst Weissleder in Menzenschwand, March 2003.

Prof. Hildegard Wittlinger
Dr. Vodder Schule
Alleestr. 30
6344 Walchsee
Austria

References

[1] Chappell D, Jacob M, Becker BF, Hofmann-Kiefer K, Conzen P, Rehm M. Expedition glycocalyx. A newly discovered "Great Barrier Reef". Anaesthesist 2008;57(10):959–969

[2] Drinker CK. The functional significance of the lymphatic system. Harvey Lecture, December 16, 1937. Bull N Y Acad Med 1938;14(5):231–251

[3] Drinker CK. The lymphatic system. Its part in regulating composition and volume of tissue fluid. The Lane Medical Lectures. Stanford, CA: Stanford University Press; 1941.

[4] Faller A, Schünke M. The Human Body. An Introduction to Structure and Function. New York, NY: Thieme; 2004.

[5] Földi M, Kubik S. Lehrbuch der Lymphologie für Mediziner, Masseure und Physiotherapeuten. 6th ed. Munich: Urban & Fischer; 2005.

[6] Herpertz U. Ödeme und Lymphdrainage—Diagnose und Therapie. 5.überarbeitete Auflage. Stuttgart: Schattauer; 2013

[7] Hutzschenreuter P, Einfeldt H, Besser S. Lymphologie für die Praxis. Stuttgart: Hippokrates; 1991.

[8] Hutzschenreuter P, Werner GT. Manual lymphatic drainage for inactivity edema with limp paresis of the arms. Manual lymphatic drainage after Dr. Vodder. 1994;4:73–76

[9] Mislin H. Vortrag bei der Wissenschaftlichen Arbeitstagung der Gesellschaft für Manuelle Lymphdrainage nach Dr. Vodder. Hamburg, 1973.

[10] Mislin H. Die Lymphdrainage als biotechnisches Problem. Erfahrungsheilkunde, Zeitschrift für die ärztliche. Praxis 1984;5:573–577

[11] Pischinger A. Das System der Grundregulation. 11th ed. Heidelberg: Haug; 2009.

[12] Schmeller W, Meier-Vollrath I. Anmerkungen zur Therapie des Lipdems. Lymphologie in Forschung und Praxis. 2006: 22–27

[13] Schmidt RF, Thews G, Lang F. Physiologie des Menschen. 28th ed. Auflage. Heidelberg: SpringerVerlag; 2000

[14] Sijmonsma J. Lymph Taping. Fysionair: Verhaag Drukkerij; 2010

[15] Van den Berg F. Angewandte Physiologie. Organsysteme verstehen. Vol 2. 2nd ed. Stuttgart: Thieme; 2005.

[16] Weissleder H, Schuchhardt C. Erkrankungen des Lymphgefäßsystems. 4th ed. Auflage. Essen: Viavital; 2006

[17] Weissleder H, Schuchhardt C. Erkrankungen des Lymphgefäßsystems. 5th ed. Auflage. Essen: Viavital; 2011

[18] Weissleder H, Schuchhardt C. Erkrankungen des Lymphgefäßsystems. 6th ed. Auflage. Köln: Viavital; 2015

[19] Winiwarter A. Die chirurgischen Krankheiten der Haut und des Zellgewebes. Stuttgart: Enke; 1892.

[20] Zoeltzer H, Suarez-Sabates C. Ultrastrukturelle Besonderheiten des Lymphendothels. LymphForsch. 2002;6(2):69–78

[21] Zoeltzer H. Funktionelle Anatomie der Lymphbildung. Lymphology 2003;36:7–25

Index

Page numbers in *italics* refer to illustrations